CW01018772

Clinician's Guide To Nuclear Medicine

Gastroenterology

Keith Harding, BSC, FRCP, FRCR
Consultant in Nuclear Medicine and
Senior Clinical Lecturer in Medicine
Dudley Road Hospital, Birmingham, UK

Philip J A Robinson, MBBS, FRCP, FRCR
Consultant Radiologist
St James's University Hospital
Leeds, UK

CHURCHILL LIVINGSTONE
EDINBURGH • LONDON • MELBOURNE • NEW YORK 1991

CHURCHILL LIVINGSTONE
Medical Division of Longman Group UK Limited

Distributed in the United States of America by
Churchill Livingstone Inc., 1560 Broadway, New York,
N.Y. 10036, and by associated companies, branches
and representatives throughout the world.

First published/Edition 1990

ISBN 0-443-04418-X

British Library Cataloguing in Publication Data
Harding, Keith
   Gastroenterology.
   1. Man. Gastrointestinal tract. Diagnosis. Applications of
   nuclear medicine
   I. Title   II. Robinson, Philip J. A (Philip Joseph Andrew)
   III. Series
   616.3307575

Library of Congress Cataloging-in-Publication Data
Harding, Keith.
   Clinicians guide to nuclear medicine – gastroenterology/Keith
Harding, Philip J.A. Robinson. – 1st ed.
      p.   cm.
   Includes index
   1. Gastrointestinal system – Radionuclide imaging.   I. Robinson,
P. J. (Philip Joseph)   II. Title.
   [DNLM: 1. Gastrointestinal Diseases – diagnosis.
2. Gastrointestinal System – radionuclide imaging.   WI 141 H263c]
RC804.R27H37   1990
616.3'307575 – dc20
DNLM/DLC
for Library of Congress

Produced by Longman Singapore Publishers Pte Ltd
Printed in Singapore

Nuclear medicine has an established place in modern medicine. The specialty is now almost 50 years old, the first clinically useful applications of the radioactive tracer method being developed in the late 1940s and early 1950s.

The scope of nuclear medicine has grown spectacularly in this period, but its nature has also altered due to the introduction and development of other imaging modalities, notably X-ray CT scanning, magnetic resonance imaging and diagnostic ultrasound. Nuclear medicine, however, remains unique in its ability to yield functionally based rather than anatomically based information.

This series of books entitled 'A Clinician's Guide to Nuclear Medicine' intends to present the clinical utility of Nuclear Medicine to all doctors, whether in general medicine/surgery or specialized disciplines, i.e. Neurology and Psychiatry, Gastroenterology, Cancer, Cardiology, Nephrourology etc.

Under the auspices of the British Nuclear Medicine Society, expert physicians from the United Kingdom have been asked to write these books. As the title of the series implies, the book should act as a guide to clinicians interested in the radioactive tracer method in their own specialty or in clinical practice. In general a series Editor has co-ordinated this development, Amersham International plc has helped to sponsor the publication of these books, and Churchill Livingstone has been appointed as Publisher for this series.

The British Nuclear Medicine Society hopes that these books will help the clinician to understand the potential and wide-ranging applications of the radioactive tracer method to Medicine in general and to clinical problem-solving in particular.

The books are well illustrated, have been purposely

Preface

designed as handbooks, and contain many useful tables and diagrams. The discussion of clinical case material is included, wherever relevant.

London, 1991   P. J. Ell

Contents

1 Introduction   1

2 The oesophagus   6

3 Gastric emptying   22

4 Hepatobiliary studies: bile reflux, jaundice
  and acute cholecystitis   31

5 Liver disease   49

6 Absorption and transit   80

7 Meckel's diverticulum   91

8 Gastrointestinal tract tumours   96

9 Inflammatory disease   105

10 Localization of gastrointestinal bleeding   116

11 The spleen   129

   Index   136

OBJECTIVES OF IMAGING

Most of the clinical manifestations of gastrointestinal disease reflect abnormal function. Dysphagia, dyspepsia, change in bowel habit, abdominal pain, gastrointestinal bleeding and jaundice are all manifestations of disturbed physiology. Whereas abnormal anatomy is usually best investigated by conventional radiology, ultrasound or computed tomography, physiological abnormalities are better defined and explored by radionuclide techniques. Magnetic resonance imaging falls somewhere between the two but is not yet sufficiently developed to play a major role in routine clinical gastroenterology. Traditionally, investigating gastrointestinal function requires intubation for sampling, or prolonged intraluminal pressure monitoring, techniques which involve a degree of discomfort to the patients. Barium studies and endoscopy, although excellent for anatomical detail, give only a very limited indication of functional disturbances. Scintigraphic studies show relatively poor anatomical detail but make their major contribution in the demonstration of abnormal function.

From the patient's point of view, radionuclide examinations are simple, requiring either a single intravenous injection or oral administration of the radionuclide. Reactions to intravenous or oral radiopharmaceuticals are exceedingly rare. Bowel preparation is not usually required and the presence of dressings or light clothing does not interfere with the examination.

In summary, the major advantages of the radionuclide procedures in investigating gastrointestinal disease are as follows:

1 The tests are non-invasive

2 In many cases quantitative assessments of disturbed function can be made
3 The radiation burden delivered to the patient is small in comparison with conventional radiological procedures
4 Because of the low radiation burden and non-invasive nature of the procedures the tests can be repeated in individual patients to follow the progress of disease or the response to treatment
5 For the same reasons normal ranges can be established in control populations

RADIATION DOSE

Absorbed radiation dose is expressed in terms of the total energy imparted to a known mass of tissue. This can be adjusted by a factor which takes into account relative biological effectiveness of the radiation involved. For gamma and beta rays this factor is 1. The unit is the sievert (Sv). Since the distribution of absorbed radiation dose is different for conventional radiography, computed tomography and radionuclide procedures it is difficult to make direct comparisons of the doses imparted by different procedures to individual body organs. An 'effective dose equivalent' (EDE) is therefore determined, and this is equivalent to the resultant whole body dose, taking into account the radiation dose and relative sensitivity of each organ (Shields & Lawson 1987). Table 1.1 lists the effective dose equivalent radiation doses typically associated with some diagnostic procedures, but it should be noted that these figures will vary with the administered activity of the radiopharmaceutical, and the presence for example of hepatic or renal failure. Some comparable risks in everyday life are quoted in Table 1.2.

APPLICATIONS OF SCINTIGRAPHY IN GASTROENTEROLOGY

Dysphagia Patients presenting with dysphagia require endoscopic or barium examination of the oesophagus. If extrinsic compression is suspected a chest radiograph and in some cases computed tomography of the thorax should be obtained. Where no anatomical obstruction is shown

Table 1.1 **Typical effective dose equivalent (EDE) from gastrointestinal investigations**

EDE	Investigations
Less than 0.5 mSv	Scintigraphic gastric emptying (^{99m}Tc), radionuclide absorption of Vit B12 studies. Chest X-ray.
0.5 – 1 mSv	Colloid liver scintigraphy, oesophageal transit test and reflux studies.
1 – 5 mSv	HIDA scintigraphy, Meckel's scintigraphy, colloid liver tomography, spleen scintigraphy, breath tests. Abdominal X-ray, CT scan, barium meal.
5 – 10 mSv	Gallium or white cell scintigraphy, labelled antibody scintigraphy, colloid or red cell scintigraphy for bleeding. Barium enema.

Table 1.2 **Everyday risks comparable with those of diagnostic nuclear medicine tests**

EDE	Equivalent risk
1 mSv	Natural background radiation level
2 mSv	Travelling 300 miles by car
5 mSv	Drinking 1 glass of wine a day for 1 year
10 mSv	Chance of a person aged 30 dying in any 2 month period Travelling 500 miles by motorcycle

scintigraphic motility studies will usually be helpful in determining the presence and progress of motility disorders (see Chapter 2).

Oesophageal reflux This is a contentious area and although it is accepted that the complications of reflux are best shown by endoscopy or double contrast barium swallow, scintigraphic methods compete with the use of prolonged intraluminal pH monitoring for detecting the presence, frequency and duration of reflux episodes (see Chapter 2).

Dyspepsia Patients with dyspeptic symptoms particularly after gastric surgery may be suffering from gastritis related to bile reflux (see Chapter 4), dumping syndromes or delayed gastric emptying (see Chapter 3).

Altered bowel habit and malabsorption Initial imaging investi-gations will include barium studies of the small bowel, large bowel enema or colonoscopy, and ultrasound or CT examination of the pancreas. If an anatomical basis for symptoms is not found, radionuclide studies of bowel transit times may be helpful. Absorption studies using labelled bile acid analogues will help to distinguish patients with diarrhoea due to bile acid malabsorption from other causes of this symptom (see Chapter 6). Vitamin B12 absorption and gastrointestinal absorption may also be examined.

Liver disease Scintigraphy is more sensitive than ultrasound or CT in the early detection of diffuse liver impairment and is in this context supplementary to biochemical tests. CT, MRI and ultrasound have better resolution for detecting small liver tumours but the first indication of occult metastatic disease can be obtained by disturbed liver blood flow patterns shown by scintigraphy. Characteristic scintigraphic appearances may point towards the diagnosis of some specific liver disorders, eg amyloid, haemangioma, Budd-Chiari syndrome (see Chapter 5).

Biliary tract disease When surgical treatment of jaundice is required then the biliary tree must be demonstrated by an anatomical method (ultrasound, CT, direct cholangiography). HIDA scintigraphy can be helpful in following the progress of liver function after biliary tract surgery or hepatic transplantation. Hepato-biliary scintigraphy can make a major contribution to the diagnosis or exclusion of acute cholecystitis or biliary atresia in children, and also provides a mechanism for the investigation of patients with acalculous biliary disease and bile leaks following surgery or trauma (see Chapter 4).

Infection, inflammation and the acute abdomen Where first-line methods are unsuccessful or inconclusive, scintigraphic demonstration of the extent of inflammatory bowel disease, the cause of pyrexia of undetermined origin, or the presence of intra-abdominal sepsis can be decisive (see Chapter 9).

Abdominal mass Detecting the presence and the extent of intra-abdominal tumours is primarily a job for ultrasound and CT scanning. However, use of radiotracer techniques for the early detection of tumour recurrence and metastases, distinguishing residual or recurrent tumour from fibrosis, and assessing anti-cancer chemotherapy are areas of potential value for scintigraphy (see Chapter 8).

Gastrointestinal bleeding In most patients upper GI endoscopy, colonoscopy or barium enema examination will show the bleeding source but a small proportion of upper GI bleeding sites, and a larger proportion of small bowel and colonic lesions, will remain occult. Scintigraphic techniques using colloid or red cells can often localize the bleeding site if used when the patient is actually bleeding (see Chapter 10). Intermittent bleeding or recurrent abdominal pain may result from a Meckel's diverticulum and this again is open to detection by a simple scintigraphic method (see Chapter 7).

REFERENCE
Shields RA, Lawson RS 1987 Effective dose equivalent. Nuclear Medicine Communications **8**: 851 – 855

CLINICAL INVESTIGATION OF OESOPHAGEAL DISEASE

Structural disease of the oesophagus is appropriately investigated by the primary methods of endoscopy and contrast radiology. The investigation of oesophageal function becomes important in two main groups of patients – firstly, those with gastro-oesophageal reflux disease, and secondly, those with dysphagia, oesophageal pain, or established neuromuscular disorders.

Reflux oesophagitis

It is now accepted that reflux per se is of little importance. The development of oesophagitis in response to reflux depends upon the frequency of reflux episodes, the volume of material retained in the oesophagus, the composition of the refluxed material (for example bile is extremely irritant), the rate of clearance of refluxed material back into the stomach, and the local resistance of the oesophageal mucosa. Prolonged ambulatory pH recording from an electrode sited within the oesophagus is the accepted reference method for documentation of the frequency and duration of reflux episodes. The scintigraphic reflux test offers a non-invasive alternative method. Comparative studies have shown a high degree of concordance between the results of pH monitoring and the results of scintigraphic reflux testing (Seibert et al 1983). In patients with endoscopically diagnosed oesophagitis, scintigraphy has been shown to be more sensitive than either pH monitoring or radiology in detecting reflux episodes (Kaul et al 1985).

Patients with reflux induced oesophagitis have a high incidence of associated motility disorder. Several studies have shown that mean transit times as measured by the scintigraphic oesophageal transit test are prolonged in the majority of patients with endoscopic evidence of active oesophagitis (Russell et al 1981; Bartlett, 1986; Kjellen et al 1987; Roland et al 1989).

Is the motility disturbance the result of reflux or its cause? The consistent observation that some patients with reflux disease have apparently normal transit times supports the view that the motility disturbance may be a primary phenomenon which predisposes to the subsequent development of oesophagitis.

Dysphagia, odynophagia and atypical chest pain

A substantial proportion of patients presenting with dysphagia will have organic obstructing lesions of the oesophagus or gastric cardia. Direct examination with double contrast barium examination or endoscopy will be diagnostic. Oesophageal function tests may have a supportive role in monitoring the results of treatment. Patients with 'transfer dysphagia' – ie difficulty in initiating the swallowing of a bolus of food resulting from spasm of the cricopharyngeus muscle, bulbar palsy, etc, are most appropriately investigated by video-fluorography which will give a qualitative indication of pharyngeal function. A substantial minority of cases will remain in which X-ray contrast studies and endoscopy appear normal. Many of these patients will have a motility disorder which can be detected by scintigraphic oesophageal transit tests. The transit test may show a characteristic adynamic pattern in achalasia or systemic sclerosis while in patients with diffuse spasm a typical incoordinate pattern is shown. The delayed transit associated with reflux disease has a less clear-cut pattern and a further group of patients will remain in whom all other tests are normal (including manometry) but scintigraphic transit is prolonged (Kjellen et al 1984).

Other oesophageal disorders

Patients with organic oesophageal obstruction have variably delayed transit times and may show almost any type of motility disorder. Most commonly the bolus is initially held up in mid or lower oesophagus but subsequently clears at a normal rate ('step-delay' pattern); in other cases of obstruction the motility may be generally diminished ('adynamic') or show a non-specific delay. About half of patients with columnar lined oesophagus show delayed transit (Karvelis et al 1987). After fundoplication for reflux disease, motility remains abnormal in a high proportion of cases but is consistently disturbed in patients complaining of post-operative dysphagia (Maddern & Jamieson 1986). Delayed transit is also fairly common after oesophageal sclerotherapy for varices and in diabetes, particularly those with other evidence of peripheral or autonomic neuropathy.

ADVANTAGES OF SCINTIGRAPHIC METHODS IN OESOPHAGEAL DISEASE

Scintigraphic methods are non-invasive and physiological, showing reflux and abnormal motility directly. In comparison with radiographic examination the radiation dose is low – a factor which may be particularly important in paediatrics. Results of scintigraphic tests are expressed numerically, and because of the non-invasive nature of the tests they can be repeated during or after treatment. The equipment and expertise required for performing these tests is easily available and their cost is relatively low. Some evidence suggests that scintigraphy is more sensitive than endoscopy in detecting abnormalities in patients with various types of oesophageal symptoms (Kjellen et al 1987).

APPLICATIONS FOR SCINTIGRAPHY IN OESOPHAGEAL DISEASE

1. Detection of abnormal oesophageal motility – scintigraphic tests have been shown to be more sensitive than endoscopy, radiography and manometry in the identification of patients with oesophageal dysmotility. The following groups of patients may fall into this category:

   (a) Patients with atypical chest pain and normal cardiological findings
   (b) Patients with dysphagia in whom endoscopy and barium examination are normal
   (c) Patients with systemic sclerosis
   (d) Patients with oesophagitis

(e) Patients with a columnar lined oesophagus

(f) Patients with post-operative or post-sclerotherapy dysphagia

(g) Diabetic patients with suspicion of autonomic neuropathy

2. Assessment of the severity of transit abnormalities in patients with established oesophageal motility disorders. This includes patients in the above groups together with those in whom the diagnosis has been made by other methods, eg patients with achalasia, diffuse oesophageal spasm and others with abnormal endoscopical or radiological findings.

3. Monitoring the effects of treatment – drugs, surgery, sclerotherapy, endoscopic dilatation, etc, on patients with established oesophageal disease.

4. Detecting the presence, frequency and duration of oesophageal reflux episodes in patients in whom gastro-oesophageal reflux disease is suspected or established, and monitoring the response to treatment.

TECHNIQUES

Oesophageal transit test (OTT)

Theory The oesophageal transit test is a method for visualizing oesophageal function, ie the transit of a swallowed bolus into the stomach. Either liquids or solids can be used but in either case the material swallowed is of physiological (food) density and the radiation dose is small compared with radiographic barium swallow. The procedure may be carried out with the patient either sitting or supine; early disturbances of motility are more likely to be detected in the supine position whereas patients with prolonged delay in oesophageal clearance (eg in achalasia) should be examined in the sitting position in order to allow gravity to assist clearing of the oesophagus. Some patients show a remarkable inconsistency in swallowing patterns and transit times between one swallow and the next; because of this it is recommended that at least six consecutive but separate swallows are recorded.

Radiopharmaceutical The technique requires only that the marker is non-absorbable and does not adhere to the surface of the oesophagus. Sulphur colloid or diethylene triamine pentacetic acid (DTPA) labelled with ^{99m}Tc are suitable markers for a liquid bolus; technetium colloid in scrambled egg is suitable for use as a solid bolus.

Preparation Patients are asked to starve for four hours (or overnight) to ensure that the stomach is empty. They should be instructed not to smoke for four hours before the examination since there is evidence that smoking may disturb oesophageal motility and promote reflux.

Acquisition The patient is instructed to swallow a 10 ml mouthful as a single bolus and then to avoid swallowing for the next 30 seconds. After one or two practice swallows with inert fluid the active swallows are carried out using 10 ml of saline flavoured with fruit juice and labelled with about 10 MBq of ^{99m}Tc colloid or DTPA. A rapid sequence of images is acquired onto computer (120 frames at 0.25 seconds each). The image acquisition is started immediately before the patient is instructed to swallow.

The above sequence is repeated twice so that initially three consecutive swallows are obtained. If activity persists in the oesophagus after the end of the acquisition period, the patient is sat up and given inert fluid to drink until the oesophagus has cleared. Three additional swallows are subsequently obtained during which the subject is asked to perform a dry swallow half-way through the acquisition period (ie at 15 seconds). If the first three swallows show gross delay in transit, the next three are conducted with the patient sitting or standing; if not, the fourth, fifth and sixth swallows are also conducted supine.

Processing – time/activity curves The oesophagus is divided along its length into three equal segments and each of these is designated as a region of interest (ROI) on the computer. A fourth ROI encompasses the whole oesophagus, and a fifth is placed on the fundus of the stomach. Time/activity curves for the whole of the oesophagus and its three sub-divisions and for the stomach

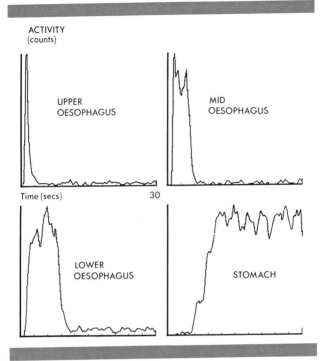

ACTIVITY
(counts)

UPPER
OESOPHAGUS

MID
OESOPHAGUS

Time (secs)   30

LOWER
OESOPHAGUS

STOMACH

Fig. 2.1 **Time/activity curves for upper, middle and lower thirds of oesophagus and for stomach in a normal subject. The time scale for all curves is 30 seconds.**

are generated from the dynamic data for each swallow (Fig. 2.1). Care must be taken in assigning the regions of interest (ROI). With the patient's head turned to one side the upper end of the oesophagus should be readily identifiable, but if there is any difficulty a radioactive marker can be placed opposite the cricoid cartilage. The ROI at the lower end of the oesophagus should not include any part of the stomach and in order to allow for diaphragmatic movement during respiration it may be necessary to exclude the lower 2 – 3 cm of the oesophagus from the regions.

Processing – functional image Appreciation of the visual data in a large series of images is simplified by the generation of a single 'condensed image' incorporating all the dynamic data into a single frame. This is achieved by compressing each frame of the acquisition along the X-axis into a single vertical profile, producing a series of one-dimensional representations of the distribution of the bolus along the length of the oesophagus. These profiles are then displayed side by side forming a functional image with the length of the oesophagus displayed on the vertical scale and time along the horizontal axis (Fig. 2.2). The progress of the bolus is charted from the mouth in the top left corner to the stomach in the bottom right (Svedberg 1982).

Results Results are expressed as mean oesophageal transit times together with a grading score based on subjective assessment of the time/activity curves and functional image.

A. *Mean transit time* Transit through the upper third of

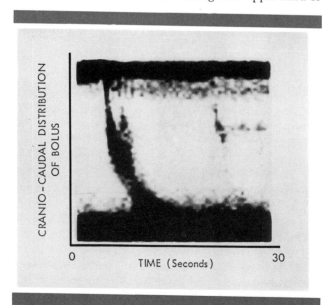

Fig. 2.2 **Functional image of a normal swallow. Time scale 30 seconds, vertical axis corresponds to the length of the oesophagus with the oral cavity at the top and gastric fundus at the bottom.**

the oesophagus normally takes about one second, about two seconds through the middle third, and about six seconds for the lower third giving an average mean transit time for the whole oesophagus in the region of eight to nine seconds.

B. *Grading system* Visual assessment allocates grades of 0 − 3, grade 0 being normal, grade 3 being a gross abnormality always involving the upper third of the oesophagus. In grade 1, the abnormality is usually confined to the lower third although there may be a minor disturbance of the mid oesophagus. With grade 2 there is a major abnormality involving the middle and lower thirds.

Abnormal patterns Abnormalities include prolongation of transit times and ineffective transmission of the swallowed bolus to the stomach, with various types of motility disturbance:

(a) reduced movement throughout the oesophagus with stasis of the bolus (adynamic pattern)
(b) fragmentation of the bolus with erratic activity throughout the oesophagus (incoordinate pattern)
(c) reverse peristalsis within the oesophagus ('intra-oesophageal reflux')
(d) temporary hold-up of the bolus in mid or lower oesophagus with subsequent clearing at normal rate (step-delay)
(e) reflux from the stomach

Examples of abnormal studies are shown in Figures 2.3 to 2.7.

Technical variations The above description relates to the use of a liquid test bolus; some workers prefer to use a solid oesophageal bolus. In this case a spoonful of scrambled egg may be given to the patient who is asked to swallow it as a single bolus after chewing. The transit times obtained are similar to those obtained with a liquid bolus as long as the patient is studied in the same position.

Patients with prolonged delay in emptying of the oesophagus should be examined in the sitting or standing

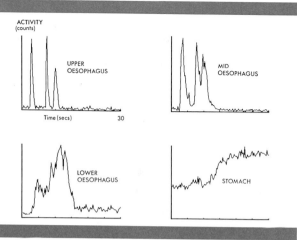

Fig. 2.3 Time/activity curves from a patient with pharyngeal incoordination leading to 'transfer dysphagia' showing fragmentation of the bolus in the upper third of the oesophagus.

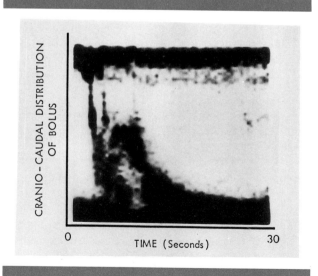

Fig. 2.4 Functional image of the swallow in the same patient as Fig. 2.3.

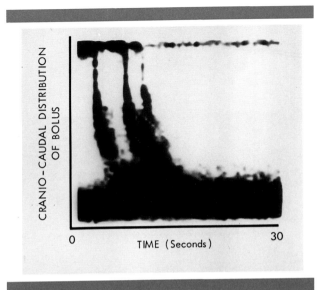

Fig. 2.5 **Functional image in patient with 'step-delay' pattern due to transitory hold up of the bolus in the middle third of the oesophagus.**

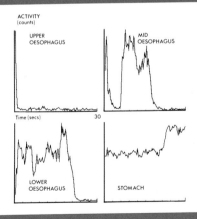

Fig. 2.6 **Time/activity curves from a patient with prolonged hold up of the bolus in middle and lower thirds of the oesophagus.**

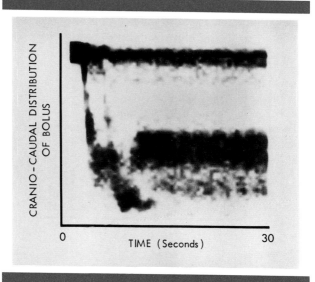

Fig. 2.7 **Functional image of a patient with reflux, showing hold up of the swallowed bolus in mid and lower oesophagus after a normal peristaltic wave has passed.**

position and even then transit times may be very long. For example in patients with achalasia, an acquisition time much longer than the usual 30 seconds may be needed in order to detect improvements in transit after treatment.

Sucralfate oesophageal study Sucralfate, an aluminium salt of polysulphated sucrose, is effective in the treatment of gastrointestinal ulceration, possibly mediating its effect by surface binding to the areas of mucosal damage. Static imaging of the gut after ingestion of sucralfate labelled with ^{99m}Tc has met with only limited success in detecting mucosal ulceration, malignancy and inflammatory bowel disease. However, substituting ^{99m}Tc-sucralfate for labelled colloid in an oesophageal motility study has been more successful in the detection and monitoring of oesophageal ulceration (Mearns et al 1989). Typically, the condensed images in patients with ulceration show retention of ^{99m}Tc-sucralfate at the site of the ulcers, whereas ^{99m}Tc-colloid is not retained. In detecting ulceration the method correlates closely with endoscopy, and could be used as an alternative to endoscopy in the follow-up of patients with established disease (Mearns et al 1989).

Binder test An alternative technique for the detection, demonstration and quantitation of gastro-oesophageal reflux involves the use of abdominal compression to provoke reflux in susceptible individuals. After filling the stomach with 500 ml of acidified orange juice labelled with ^{99m}Tc-colloid or DTPA, an abdominal binder incorporating a broad sphygmomanometer cuff is inflated in steps of 20 mm Hg from zero to 100 mm Hg. At each level of pressure a gamma camera image of the lower oesophagus and stomach is obtained. Radioactivity appearing in the oesophagus in increasing quantities as the binder pressure rises is taken as evidence of reflux (Fig. 2.8). By measuring the relative count rates from oesophagus and stomach a 'reflux index' can be calculated.

Although some workers have found this test to be a sensitive and accurate indicator of reflux disease (Fisher et al 1976) in other hands it has been less reliable. Increasing the intra-abdominal pressure may herniate the stomach into the chest in patients with a lax hiatus, while in other cases reflux is unrelated to thoraco-abdominal pressure gradients. Good correlation between a positive binder test and endoscopic or histological evidence of oesophagitis has not been consistently found.

Physiological oesophageal reflux test

Theory This is a test to detect gastro-oesophageal reflux under physiological circumstances. The object of the test is to detect not only the existence of reflux episodes but their frequency, duration (ie the rate of clearance back into the stomach) and also the volume of material refluxed. The test is performed by filling the stomach with a labelled marker then positioning the gamma camera over the stomach and oesophagus to chart the progress of the labelled material over a prolonged period; 40 – 60 minutes has been shown to be an adequate sampling period for this purpose.

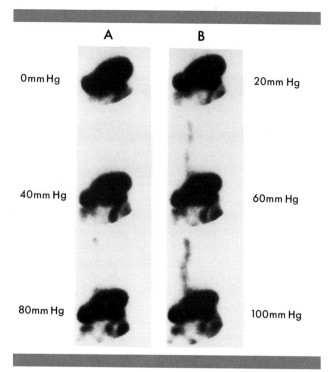

Fig. 2.8 **Binder test: 30 second images of the chest and upper abdomen with successive increases in abdominal binder pressure. Reflux visible in the oesophagus at the higher pressures.**

Radiopharmaceutical As with the transit test, the marker needs to be non-absorbable and also be unaffected by gastric enzymes and acid. The test meal is acidified in order to enhance oesophageal symptoms in the event that reflux episodes were to occur.

Acquisition The patient drinks 500 ml of the test meal which is made up of equal volumes of orange juice and N/10 hydrochloric acid to which has been added 20 MBq of ^{99m}Tc-labelled colloid or diethylene triamine pentacetic acid (DTPA).

After ingesting the test meal, the patient then drinks

additional unlabelled liquid until the residual activity in the oesophagus has been cleared into the stomach. If the reflux test is performed immediately after the transit test, no additional radioactivity needs to be given; an inert test meal will mix adequately with residual radioactivity in the stomach.

The patient is positioned semi-recumbent with the gamma camera centred over the stomach and lower oesophagus. Images are obtained at 20-second intervals for 40 minutes.

Processing Time/activity curves are obtained by setting regions of interest over the stomach, the oesophagus, and an area of background (lung) activity. The count rate over the oesophagus is usually extremely low and a background region is helpful to act as a control for any spurious peaks in count rate, caused by movement of the patient or by detection of transient radioactivity from sources outside the patient. In order to distinguish genuine episodes of reflux from statistical fluctuations in the oesophageal time/activity curve due to quantum noise, a computer program is used to highlight those points or groups of points which are more than three standard deviations above neighbouring points on the curve (Fig. 2.9).

Results Results are expressed in terms of the number of

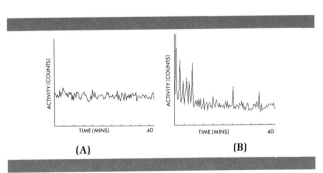

Fig. 2.9 **Time/activity curves from the oesophagus over 40 minutes. A, Normal patient showing fluctuations due to statistical noise. B, Multiple episodes of reflux of short duration.**

reflux episodes occurring during the observation period and the duration of each episode. An arbitrary normal guideline is that no more than one episode of reflux should occur during a 40 minute period; the episode should last no more than 20 seconds (one or two frames of data). With prolonged episodes of reflux, the area under the 'spike' in the curve is proportional to the product of the volume of material refluxed and the duration of the episode, both relevant factors in the pathogenesis of oesophagitis.

Milk scan Reflux in infants can be investigated by adding [99mTc] colloid or DTPA to a normal milk feed then placing the infant prone over a gamma camera for 60 minutes of acquisition. Sensitivity of detection of reflux by this approach is superior to that of barium examination.

Late images of the chest can be obtained in infants suspected of recurrent pulmonary aspiration of food; this technique occasionally shows spill-over of the labelled feed into the lungs but is not sensitive enough to rule out aspiration if a negative result is obtained.

REFERENCES

Bartlett RJV 1986 Scintigraphy of the oesophagus. In: PJ Robinson (ed) Nuclear gastroenterology, Churchill Livingstone, Edinburgh, pp. 12 – 14

Fisher RS, Malmud LS, Roberts GS, Lobis IF 1976 Gastroesophageal scintiscanning to detect and quantitate GE reflux. Gastroenterology **70**: 301 – 308

Karvelis KC, Drane WE, Johnson DA, Silverman ED 1987 Barrett esophagus: decreased esophageal clearance shown by radionuclide esophageal scintigraphy. Radiology **162**: 97 – 99

Kaul B, Petersen H, Grette K, Erichsen H, Myrvold HE 1985 Scintigraphy, pH measurement, and radiography in the evaluation of gastroesophageal reflux. Scandinavian Journal of Gastroenterology **20**: 289 – 294

Kjellen G, Svedberg JB, Tibbling L 1984 Solid bolus transit by oesophageal scintigraphy in patients with dysphagia and normal manometry and radiography. Digestive Diseases & Sciences **29**: 1 – 5

Kjellen G, Andersson P, Sandstrom S 1987 Esophageal scintigraphy: a comparison with esophagoscopy. Scandinavian Journal of Gastroenterology 22: 75 – 81

Maddern GJ, Jamieson GG 1986 Oesophageal emptying in patients with gastro-oesophageal reflux. British Journal of Surgery 73: 615 – 617

Mearns AJ, Hart GC, Cox JA 1989 Dynamic radionuclide imaging with ^{99m}T-sucralfate in the detection of oesophageal ulceration. Gut 30: 1256 – 1259

Roland J, Peters O, Piepsz A, Devis G, Jonckheer M, Ham HR 1989 Evaluation of oesophageal transit in patients with minor peptic oesophagitis. Nuclear Medicine Communications 10: 161 – 165

Russell COH, Pope CE, Gannon RM, Allen FD, Velasco N, Hill LD 1981 Does surgery correct oesophageal motor dysfunction in gastroesophageal reflux? Annals of Surgery 194: 290 – 296

Seibert JJ, Byrne WJ, Euler AR, Latture A, Leach M, Campbell M 1983 Gastroesophageal reflux – the acid test: scintigraphy or the pH probe? American Journal of Roentgenology 104: 1087 – 1090

Svedberg JB 1982 The bolus transport diagram: a functional display method applied to oesophageal studies. Clinical Physics & Physiological Measurement 3: 267 – 272

3 | Gastric Emptying

Abnormalities of gastric emptying occur most often after surgical treatment for peptic ulceration, but as drug therapy has become more successful surgery is less often performed than previously. In a large series of patients Goligher et al (1978) showed that the symptoms of dumping or stasis were not uncommon following gastric surgery (Table 3.1).

Table 3.1 **Percentage incidence of symptoms after gastric surgery**

Surgery	Dumping	Stasis
Subtotal gastrectomy	22	6
Vagotomy and gastroenterostomy	18	4
Vagotomy and pyloroplasty	12	4
Vagotomy and antrectomy	9	10
Proximal gastric vagotomy	1	9

After Goligher et al 1978

PROBLEMS AFTER GASTRIC SURGERY

Dumping syndrome
The patient complains of faintness which may be accompanied by dizziness, weakness, palpitation, sweating and pallor. Some patients also complain of abdominal discomfort, borborygmi, and epigastric fullness. Early dumping symptoms generally occur within 30 minutes of the patient taking a meal, and are due to rapid gastric emptying of part of the meal into the small intestine, and are associated with a fall in the plasma volume. Late

dumping symptoms occur 1 – 2 hours after a meal and are due to reactive hypoglycaemia occurring when the meal empties rapidly into the small intestine. Symptoms include pallor, sweating, weakness, tremor and fainting, and are relieved by sugar.

Diarrhoea

Symptoms of diarrhoea early after gastric surgery are relatively common. In a small percentage of these, symptoms persist due to the osmotic effect of food in the duodenum. Rarely the cause of the diarrhoea is a Zollinger-Ellison syndrome which is due to a gastrin secreting tumour.

Gastric stasis

Patients with gastric stasis complain of feeling full after meals, nausea, and may vomit food a long time after a meal has been taken.

The role of scintigraphy

Most clinical problems involving the stomach are resolved by endoscopy with biopsy, or barium examination. Delayed gastric emptying may be apparent using either of these techniques because of residual food in the stomach, and using a barium examination it is possible to provide a rough estimate of emptying. However, barium is not a physiological need. Radionuclide gastric emptying studies allow a relatively normal meal to be used and frequent observations made of the amount of meal remaining in the stomach. Gastric emptying studies are not required after surgery in all patients, and should only be undertaken in those with troublesome symptoms. It is however important to confirm that there is an abnormality of gastric emptying before further surgery for dumping or stasis is undertaken.

Differentiating the neurotic from those with impairment of gastric emptying may be very difficult, since many symptoms such as faintness, abdominal discomfort, dizziness and diarrhoea are common in functional gastric disorders. Results of re-operation because of persistent pain are inevitably poor in such patients, and a normal gastric emptying study will identify a group who do not need further surgery. Donovan et al (1974) have shown that abnormalities of gastric emptying improve over the period of one year following operation, so whenever possible re-operation should be avoided over this period even if an abnormality of gastric emptying can be demonstrated.

Other indications for gastric emptying studies

Gastric emptying studies may be useful in other groups of patients. In diabetics they may be helpful in identifying abnormal patterns of emptying and the diet can be modified accordingly. Obese patients usually show rapid gastric emptying. In severe obesity where gastric plication operation is required, gastric emptying studies may be helpful in assessing emptying after surgery. A number of drugs delay gastric emptying and these include anticholinergics, opiates, and tricylic antidepressants. Rarely it may be necessary to confirm problems in gastric emptying with such patients.

Technique

Theory The patient is given a meal labelled with a radioactive tracer and the amount of that tracer remaining in the stomach is determined at frequent intervals using a gamma camera. It should be noted that this test does not measure the volume of the stomach since the gastric secretions are not radioactive. There is a wide variation in techniques used to measure gastric emptying and express the results. The position in which the study is performed is not standardized but it is clear that particularly after vagotomy gastric emptying is gravity dependent (McKelvey 1970) so that the patient should be either sitting or standing, rather than lying.

The patient's perception Gastric emptying studies are not unpleasant from the patient's point of view. Both a liquid and a solid meal are generally required and these may be given as one meal containing two different radioactive markers or on two separate days. Patients need to starve for four hours prior to the study and because smoking delays gastric emptying it should be avoided during this period. Drugs which affect gastric emptying (see above) should be stopped for 24 hours when the study is required to assess emptying after surgery.

In departments where studies are performed in a sitting position, women should be asked to wear trousers as the patient has to sit with their legs wide apart if the gamma camera is to be positioned correctly.

During the study the patient eats a meal and if they can only take small quantities of food it is important to inform the nuclear medicine department so that the technique can be modified accordingly.

Radiopharmaceutical The liquid meal may be labelled with ^{99m}Tc, ^{111}In or ^{113m}In DTPA (diethylene-triamine pentacetic acid). This marker is not absorbed nor does it stick to the gastric mucus or mucosa. The author uses DTPA as a label for 10% dextrose solution in liquid gastric emptying studies, and as semi-solid meal we use meat, potatoes, peas and milk. For solid meals others have used resins, strips of absorbent paper coated with perspex cement, scrambled egg, and bran (Donovan & Harding 1986). An elegant technique has been described in which a chicken is given the radioactive sulphur colloid, the chicken is killed, and the liver incorporated into a meal. While the stability of the label is certain using this method it is quite unnecessary for clinical gastric emptying studies. Whatever meal is chosen it is important that its composition is kept the same for all studies, as gastric emptying depends upon the volume of the meal, calorific content and the size of particles in the meal.

Data acquisition Because the meal moves forward in the abdomen as the stomach empties, it is necessary with low energy radionuclides (^{99m}Tc or ^{111}In) to take alternative anterior and posterior images in order to correct for change in detection efficiency. With higher energy ra-diopharmaceuticals such as ^{113m}In this problem is much smaller (Harding & Donovan 1988) and anterior views only are sufficient.

Images of the stomach are taken at frequent intervals

(1 – 5 min) during the course of emptying of the meal. For liquid meals, a study duration of 40 minutes is sufficient, but with solid meals a longer study of 90 minutes is generally required.

Processing the data It may be necessary to correct the data (Harding & Donovan 1988) for patient movement, down scatter of higher energy photons into lower energy window where a dual isotope technique is used, and scattered counts being detected outside the stomach area. Results of solid meal emptying are usually expressed as the $t^1/_2$ of the meal calculated by assuming an exponential fall in counts and applying a 'best fit' line to the data. With liquid meals it has been argued that the curve is not exponential but more nearly linear. In reality differences between linear and exponential fit are small.

The $t^1/_2$ by itself can be misleading. In patients with severe dumping much of the meal may leave the stomach before peak counts occur, and the remainder of the meal leaves slowly with a long $t^1/_2$. It is important therefore to relate counts in the stomach to the volume of meal administered so that this early emptying can be detected. Results are expressed as the peak volume in the stomach and the $t^1/_2$. The peak volume of the liquid meal is a particularly useful parameter in assessing dumping, and a $t^1/_2$ of the solid meal more discriminating for detection of stasis.

Normal results Because of the wide variety of techniques available, each department should determine its own normal range. A typical liquid meal peak volume is 330 ml (SD 50 ml) in patients given a 400 ml meal. Using a semi-solid meal of meat, potatoes and peas with milk the normal $t^1/_2$ is 40 minutes (Fig. 3.1 A, B) with a typical range of 28 – 80 (the standard deviation is not quoted as the $t^1/_2$ is not normally distributed). It is important in calculating the $t^1/_2$ not to include data points when the volume of the meal remaining in the stomach is small, that is less than 25% of the administered volume (Harding & Donovan 1988). Beyond this point errors are large.

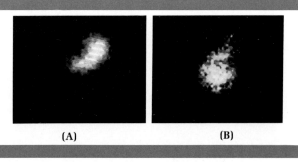

(A)   (B)

Fig. 3.1 **Normal gastric emptying study. The shape of the stomach is evident at 5 min (A) and by 50 min (B) approximately half of the meal has emptied.**

Criteria of abnormality Symptoms of dumping occur in patients who have peak liquid meal volumes in the stomach of less than 240 ml (400 ml meal), but interestingly only a third of patients with such low peak volumes are symptomatic (Fig. 3.2). Stasis is associated with a $t^1/_2$ of the solid meal greater than 150 minutes (Fig. 3.3), and in this case only half of the patients with such delayed emptying will be symptomatic.

Dosimetry For 12 MBq [113m]In or 40 MBq ^{99m}Tc the EDE is low at 0.3 mSv, but with [111]In (12 MBq) somewhat greater at 4 mSv.

Findings in specific disorders Typical findings after ulcer surgery are shown in Table 3.2 (Donovan & Harding 1986). The older Polya gastrectomy generally results in a low liquid meal peak volume (mean 205 ml) and a considerable delay in emptying ($t^1/_2$ 21 – 323 min) for the semi-solid meal. The more selective truncal vagotomy upsets gastric emptying less, and the least change from normal is found after a highly selective proximal gastric vagotomy.

Problems with the technique In those with large stomachs, or if the stomach lies in the pelvis, there are substantial errors in attempting to measure gastric emptying because

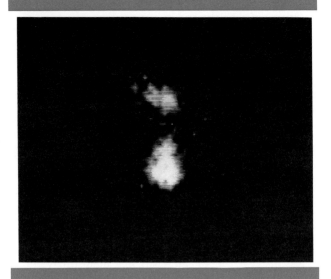

Fig. 3.2 **Dumping. At 5 min after ingestion the majority of the meal has left the stomach.**

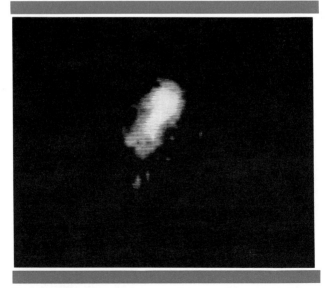

Fig. 3.3 **Stasis. The 90 min stomach image shows minimal emptying.**

Table 3.2 **Result of gastric emptying after surgery for duodenal ulcer**

	Liquid meal		Solid meal	
	peak volume (ml)	median (SD)	t$^{1}/_{2}$ min	median (20 – 80%)
Normal	330	(50)	40	(28 – 80)
PGV	280	(60)	40	(24 – 80)
TV + P	235	(70)	36	(12 – 176)
Polya	205	(75)	49	(21 – 323)
Symptoms	<240		>150	
Proportion symptomatic	1:3		1:2	

PGV, Proximal gastric vagotomy; TV+P, Truneal vagotomy and pyloroplasty; Polya, Polya gastrectomy

of overlap of the meal in the stomach and the remainder of the bowel (Table 3.3). In such patients it is necessary to use an alternative technique such as naso-intubation and intermittent sampling of the gastric contents (Wolverson et al 1982).

Table 3.3 **Peak volume (ml) of meal in the stomach determined by two methods in control and gastric ulcer patients. Corresponding stomach areas on planar images (arbitrary units)**

Peak volume	Control (SD)		Gastric ulcer (SD)	
Camera	133	(36)	236	(32)
Aspiration	118	(30)	165	(66)
Stomach area	898	(296)	1265	(329)

REFERENCES
Donovan IA, Keighley MRB, Griffin DW et al 1974 The

association of duodeno-gastric reflux with dumping and gastric retention. British Journal of Surgery **63**: 34 – 35

Donovan IA, Harding LK 1986 Gastric Emptying. In: Robinson PJ (ed) Nuclear gastroenterology. Churchill Livingstone, Edinburgh pp. 24 – 35

Goligher JC, Hill GL, Kerry TE et al 1978 Proximal gastric vagotomy without drainage for duodenal ulcer: results after 5 – 8 years. British Journal of Surgery **65**: 145 – 151

Harding LK, Donovan IA 1988 Gastric emptying: gastro-oesophageal reflux. In: Rhys Davies E, Thomas WEG (eds), Nuclear Medicine – Applications to Surgery, Castle House Publications, Tunbridge Wells pp. 42 – 51

McKelvey STD 1970 Gastric incontinence and post vagotomy diarrhoea. British Journal of Surgery **57**: 741 – 747

Wolverson RL, Harding LK, Alexander-Williams J, Donovan IA, Derges SB, Sorgi M 1982 Improvement of the double sampling dye dilution technique for measuring gastric emptying. Gastro-enterology **82**: p. 1213

BILE REFLUX

Introduction

Two hundred years ago John Hunter, the eminent Scottish anatomist and surgeon, suggested that bile in the stomach caused nausea. Dispute over the relevance of bile in dyspepsia has continued since then, but when imino diacetic acid (HIDA) derivatives became generally available 12 years ago it seemed that the problems might be resolved. HIDA derivatives are labelled with ^{99m}Tc so that image quality is high. They clear the blood pool rapidly after intravenous injection and are excreted into the bile. Detection of bile reflux requires careful attention to technique, and some experience in interpreting the images.

Role of scintigraphy

Post peptic ulcer surgery Operations for peptic ulcer are much less common than they were a few years ago, because effective medical treatment for duodenal and gastric ulcer is now available. In addition endoscopy has improved diagnostic accuracy.

After peptic ulcer surgery some patients continue to have symptoms, even after excluding those with recurrent ulceration or biliary tract disease. Bile reflux should be considered as a possible explanation for the symptoms in such patients. It is more common after an operation in which the anatomy of the pylorus has been altered, and after proximal gastric vagotomy (Mosimann et al 1984) is no more frequent than in a control population. The main features of bile reflux are bile vomiting, epigastric pain and heartburn, and these can be relieved by a Roux-en-Y anastomosis or an isoperistaltic jejunal interposition. These operations reduce the amount of reflux with an improvement in the patient's symptoms. However it is important to perform a bile reflux study in any patient where bile reflux is being considered as a cause for their symptoms, and if reflux cannot be provoked with cholecystokinin (CCK) then another cause for their symptoms, for example rapid gastric emptying, should be considered (Harding & Donovan 1986).

Oesophageal reflux after total gastrectomy Patients who have had gastrectomy for gastric cancer may have bile reflux into the oesophagus, with the production of ulcerative oesophagitis. Reflux can be demonstrated using a bile reflux test, and we have shown that the occurrence of reflux is related to the length of the Roux-en-Y loop. Patients who refluxed had loops less than 35 cm long and no case of reflux occurred in a patient with a loop longer than this. All loops used in Roux-en-Y reconstruction should be 50 cm long.

Flatulent dyspepsia Cholecystectomy is a common operation and there is a proportion of patients after surgery who continue to complain of flatulence, heartburn, abdominal distension and right upper quadrant pain. The question arises as to whether the gallstones were coincidental and the patient had a different cause for their symptoms. Johnson (1972) suggested that there was a correlation between 'flatulent' or 'gallstone' dyspepsia and pyloric regurgitation. In a previous paper (Johnson 1971) he had studied 108 patients undergoing cholecystectomy and found that 83% had flatulent dyspepsia: only 46% were symptom free after the operation. However Harding et al (1986) have shown the same incidence and amount of reflux in patients with gallstones whether or not they had flatulent dyspepsia. Controversy continues but in those whose symptoms persist after surgery it is important to consider other causes. These include oesophagitis or peptic ulcer, the complications of upper abdominal surgery such as infection, adhesions or intraduct stones, and finally strictures or sphincter of Oddi stenosis. Only when these have been eliminated should bile reflux be considered as a cause of the symptoms and this should be demonstrated scintigraphically.

Technique

Theory The HIDA molecule is related to lignocaine, is excreted unchanged by the liver, and undergoes no enterohepatic circulation. It is ideal therefore to examine problems of bile kinetics including bile reflux.

Radiopharmaceutical Using diethyl HIDA Harding et al (1984) showed that only 5% of the radiopharmaceutical remained in the blood stream 30 minutes after injection, and that the peak biliary excretion occurred at 45 – 60 minutes. They also established a close correlation between the amount of HIDA and bile acid in the stomach.

Other HIDA derivatives behave somewhat differently in terms of the rate of blood clearance, time of excretion and proportion of the radiopharmaceutical excreted by the kidneys. The higher derivatives of HIDA (for example parabutyl or Iodo HIDA) are excreted at higher bilirubin levels (Harding & Donovan 1986), and should be used in jaundiced patients.

The patient's perception From the patient's point of view the main problem with the test is discomfort in lying still during the course of the study which may last over $1\frac{1}{2}$ hr. No nasogastric intubation is required, and the only difficulty which may arise is if the patient is given CCK to contract the gallbladder. Some patients experience pain with the CCK, and may develop severe colic or hypotension. Hydrocortisone should be available at the time of the injection.

Acquisition Various protocols have been used (Harding & Donovan 1986). A typical one is described.

After an overnight fast patients are given 75 MBq [99mTc] diethyl HIDA intravenously. After 20 minutes they are positioned under a large field of view gamma camera and at 30 minutes imaging begins. In order to take into account any patient movement [57Co] markers are placed on the anterior iliac crests. Computer frames are collected at intervals of 30 seconds and analogue images each 2 minutes. At 45 minutes patients are given either 70 units CCK by slow intravenous injection, or a liquid fatty meal of 370 kilocalories containing 20 g of fat. At the end of the study 200 ml of water is given through a straw to diffuse any activity in the stomach, and prove therefore that it is not in loops of bowel, and after further images, 6 – 8 MBq of ^{99m}Tc HIDA in 100 ml of water is given to outline the stomach.

Normal appearance The position of the stomach can be compared with any possible area of reflux noticed on the previous images, using the ^{57}Co markers on the anterior iliac crests for accurate superimposition (Fig. 4.1 A, B).

Studying the sequence of images obtained may also be helpful in deciding if activity is present in the stomach. However a varying proportion of normal subjects will show reflux, depending on the technique used. With the protocol described 12% of symptomless controls reflux after a fatty meal, and 45% after CCK.

Abnormal appearances Various criteria have been used to decide if a study is reflux positive or not (Fig. 4.2 A, B). Using the technique described above reflux was considered

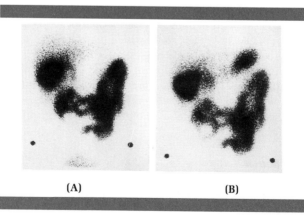

(A)   (B)

Fig. 4.1 **A, At the end of a bile reflux study there is HIDA in a high loop of bowel. B, The ^{99m}Tc drink confirms the position of the stomach. Note the ^{57}Co markers on the anterior iliac crests.**

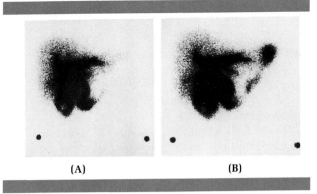

(A)   (B)

Fig. 4.2 **A, Reflux study at 46 minutes after injection of the HIDA. B, At 48 minutes there is bile influx into the stomach.**

present if it occurred in three successive two minute images. In practice, reflux usually lasts for much longer than this, as it clears by gastric emptying. The brief episodes of reflux into the distal stomach which can be identified on barium examination are not detected by the HIDA technique.

Dosimetry The EDE for 60 – 80 MBq of HIDA is 1.5 mSv, with the gallbladder, which is the critical organ, receiving 7 mGy.

Sensitivity Using the technique described above Sorgi et al (1984) showed that the test is sensitive to 1% of the amount of administered HIDA in the stomach. They also examined reproducibility by studying patients twice in the same week, and found that the same reflux pattern occurred in only 75%. In view of the known sensitivity of the test this almost certainly represents day-to-day variation in the amount of reflux.

Choice of imaging technique An isotope test provides the only available way of demonstrating enterogastric reflux of bile both quantitatively and physiologically. Reflux of bile into the stomach is often observed at gastroscopy, but the significance of this is uncertain because the large tube in the stomach may induce reflux. Conventional naso-gastric tubes however have been shown not to provoke reflux.

J A U N D I C E

Introduction

As imaging techniques have developed the method of investigation of jaundice has altered. The major advance has been in the improved resolution of ultrasound, and this now should be the first investigation of the jaundiced patient. While dilated ducts indicate an obstructive cause for the jaundice, it is important to demonstrate the site and nature of the obstruction and this may require other imaging techniques. However the emphasis is now changing to try and detect those patients with partial or intermittent bile obstruction where the bile duct diameter is normal.

Imaging tests – the role of scintigraphy

Using conventional ultrasound apparatus the gallbladder is easily visualized and any stones detected. Normal intrahepatic ducts cannot be identified. In approximately two-thirds of cases of jaundice the site of the obstruction can be determined using ultrasound. Computerized tomography (CT) is complementary to ultrasound, especially in those with intestinal gas which prevents ultrasound examination. It is possible with CT to assess the bile ducts, gallbladder and often the level of the obstruction, although as with ultrasound normal calibre ducts cannot be demonstrated.

In those with severely dilated ducts percutaneous transhepatic cholangiography will demonstrate the detailed anatomy of the biliary tree and the site of the obstruction. However it should not be used in patients who have abnormally long prothrombin times, or low platelet counts. When the block is in the distal end of the bile duct or pancreas, endoscopy with retrograde cholangiopancreatography (ERCP) is particularly useful to remove stones by sphincterotomy. Passage of stents into malignant obstruction is also a useful procedure which improves the quality of life.

The use of scintigraphy in demonstrating the cystic duct obstruction of acute cholecystitis is described later. It is also an important test in young children with obstructive jaundice where biliary atresia is being considered. Thirdly, in post-operative patients biliary leaks may be demonstrated non-invasively, and without increasing pressure in the biliary system by injection of radiographic contrast media. Finally there is the rare patient where the spectrum of diagnostic tests has failed to find a cause for jaundice. This includes occasional patients with a marked bleeding tendency or with a history of severe reactions to contrast media. The protocol is the same as that in post-operative patients.

BILIARY ATRESIA

While there are several causes of conjugated hyperbilirubinaemia in the neonatal period the main clinical problem arises in differentiating neonatal hepatitis and biliary atresia. The latter is rare but its diagnosis important. Jaundice usually becomes apparent within 2 or 3 weeks of birth. The Kasai operation, which aims to create drainage of bile into the bowel, achieves the best results if it is performed during the first three months of life. Because of the small size of the liver and bile ducts, ultrasound and other imaging tests are particularly difficult in this group of patients, although the presence of a normal gallbladder virtually rules out the diagnosis of atresia. Biopsy of the liver is often helpful but not always definitive.

Role of scintigraphy

Scintigraphy is part of the spectrum of investigations necessary to establish a diagnosis of biliary atresia. However images have to be taken for up to 24 hours because in some cases of neonatal hepatitis excretion of the HIDA is slow.

Method

Theory The children are pre-treated with oral phenobarbitone 5 mg/kg for 3 – 5 days prior to the study. This enhances excretion of HIDA by inducing the liver enzymes. Excretion of HIDA into the bowel excludes the diagnosis of biliary atresia.

Acquisition Patient movement is less if neonates are imaged prone. Diisopropyl-HIDA is given in proportion to the child's weight or surface area, based on a corresponding adult dose of 150 MBq. Images are taken at 15 minute intervals for 1 hour, and hourly up to 4 hours. If no excretion has occurred at 24 hours images on the following day are necessary.

Scintigraphic appearances Examples of early excretion in a case of neonatal hepatitis, and failure to excrete the HIDA in the case of biliary atresia are shown in Figures 4.3 and 4.4.

Problems with the test The poor quality of images obtained at 24 hours, urinary excretion, and urine on nappies may cause problems in interpreting the images. The latter problem may resolved by a clean nappy and taking a

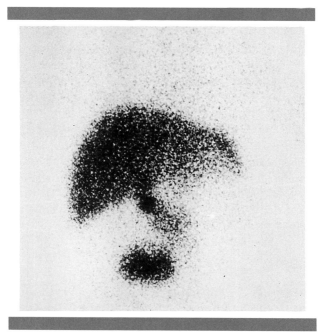

Fig. 4.3 **Excretion of HIDA into the bowel at 24 minutes in a case of neonatal hepatitis.**

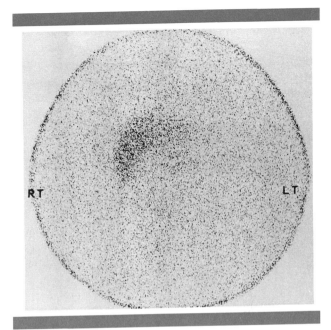

Fig. 4.4 **Failure to excrete the HIDA in a case of biliary atresia. The image is of poor quality as it is taken 24 hr after injection.**

lateral view if difficulties still exist. However in most children who are going to show excretion, this has occurred by 2 hours and the test can be terminated.

Sensitivity Dick & Mowat (1986) have reported an accuracy of 90%. The same group have suggested that a liver-to-heart ratio between $2\frac{1}{2}$ and 10 minutes post injection of HIDA greater than 5 excludes biliary atresia. Others (Charlton et al 1988) have failed to confirm this and consider it important therefore to image up to 24 hours.

POST-OPERATIVE PATIENTS

Introduction

Complications following surgery of the biliary tract include retained stones and biliary leaks. Following liver transplant, prolongation of jaundice may be due to biliary obstruction, rejection, infection, or vascular problems (Fig. 4.5 A, B).

Role of scintigraphy Most of the complications of biliary surgery can be diagnosed with ultrasound and endoscopy with ERCP. Sometimes CT or percutaneous cholangiograms are required but in a difficult case scintigraphy may be useful. It will detect biliary obstruction for example due to retained stones, and also biliary leaks (Figs. 4.6 A, B; 4.7 A, B).

After liver transplant it is traditional to leave a t-tube in the bile duct so that cholangiography may be performed. However t-tube cholangiograms may cause septicaemia so prophylactic antibiotics are required, and in any case the t-tube may not adequately show the intrahepatic bile ducts. A HIDA study may be used, especially in children where the bile ducts are small.

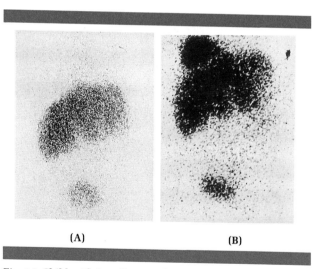

(A)   (B)

Fig. 4.5 **Child with jaundice post liver transplant. An initial HIDA study (A) showed poor liver uptake and a cold area in the upper pole of the right lobe. A subsequent image (B) shows that bile has leaked into the abscess cavity beneath the diaphragm.**

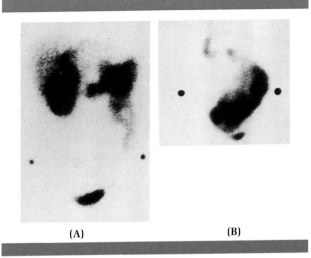

(A)   (B)

Fig. 4.6 **A, Collection of bile behind the duodenum. Some bile has drained normally into the bowel. B, Post repair of bile leak the majority of the bile has passed into the bowel at the same time (78 minutes) post injection. (Note HIDA present in the bladder.)**

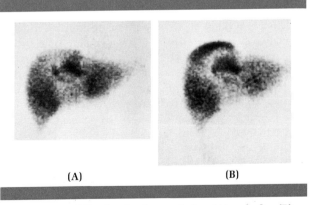

(A)   (B)

Fig. 4.7 **HIDA study showing images before (A) and after (B) leakage of bile into the subphrenic space.**

Radiopharmaceutical In those without jaundice, or those mildly jaundiced, diisopropyl HIDA may be used. In jaundiced patients it is advisable to use one of the higher forms of HIDA such as Iodo HIDA which is excreted at higher bilirubin levels.

Acquisition Because it may be important to visualize the bile ducts in detail in the post-operative patient, 2-minute images up to 30 minutes after injection are recommended. Thereafter hourly images are taken up to 4 – 6 hours, and a final one at 24 hours.

Appearances Excretion into the bowel normally occurs by 30 minutes. It is important to look for abnormal accumulation of HIDA due to a biliary leak. Even if excretion is prompt, pooling in the bile ducts or in the secondary bile ducts is indicative of obstruction.

Finally HIDA may reveal areas of the liver where blood supply is compromised in those who have had liver transplants.

Dosimetry Dosimetry is the same as for biliary atresia.

A C U T E   C H O L E C Y S T I T I S

Incidence and presentation

Gallstones develop in a proportion of adults variously estimated at between 10 and 30%. Acute cholecystitis develops in a minority of these, but is extremely rare in patients without gallstones. The major factor predisposing to the development of acute cholecystitis is stasis of bile in the gall bladder. Defective emptying promotes chemical injury to the gall bladder mucosa from constant exposure to concentrated bile, and once stones have been formed the possibility of cystic duct obstruction becomes much more likely. Almost all patients with acute cholecystitis have gallstones obstructing the cystic duct, but in a minority the duct is obstructed by other causes including stricture, kinking, torsion, intussusception of polyps, external pressure by malignant nodes and gall bladder carcinoma. With increasing distension, the blood supply to the gall bladder is reduced and subsequent bacterial infection becomes increasingly likely. Typical clinical presentation is with right upper quadrant pain, nausea and vomiting, pyrexia, leucocytosis and local tenderness over the gall bladder area. However, similar clinical findings may be present in patients with subhepatic or subphrenic infections, acute hepatitis or liver abscess, right sided pyelonephritis or diverticulitis, retrocaecal appendix, and penetrating or perforated duodenal ulcer. In elderly patients the diagnosis may be particularly difficult since some cases may show no localizing features in spite of severe biliary tract infection or even gangrene of the gall bladder.

Rationale for investigation

It has been estimated that about one-third of patients presenting with the above clinical picture will actually have acute cholecystitis (Laing et al 1981). If we accept that about 20% of adult patients have gallstones, one in five of the patients presenting with other acute right upper quadrant pathologies will also have gallstones. This means that a substantial minority (a quarter to a third) of patients with gallstones who present with the clinical features of acute cholecystitis will actually have a different pathology responsible for their illness. Since cholecystectomy remains the final common pathway for most patients presenting with acute cholecystitis, and the morbidity of biliary tract surgery is not trivial, a strong case exists for establishing a diagnosis as firmly as possible before proceeding to surgery.

There is now no place for radiographic contrast examinations of the biliary tract in this condition. The oral cholecystogram is inappropriate and unreliable in the acutely ill patient, while intravenous cholangiography is an unsatisfactory examination from many points of view and should be regarded as obsolete. Ultrasound scanning is both sensitive and reliable in the detection of stones in the gall bladder but the ultrasonic features of acute cholecystitis are less consistent and less specific. Thickening of the gall bladder wall can be seen in chronic cholecystitis; distension of the gall bladder needs to be gross before it can be confidently recognised as abnormal; and the sonolucent layer seen in the gall bladder wall of patients with inflammatory disease is also found in gall bladder oedema due to heart failure, cirrhosis or cholangitis.

The only technique which reliably demonstrates cystic duct obstruction is hepato-biliary scintigraphy. As mentioned above, the vast majority of patients with acute cholecystitis have physical obstruction of the cystic duct. In the small proportion of patients in whom the cystic duct is found not to be mechanically obstructed at surgery, stasis of bile still plays a major role in the genesis of acute cholecystitis and in these cases there appears to be functional obstruction. The morbidity and mortality from acute acalculous cholecystitis is considerably higher than in patients with gallstone obstruction of the cystic duct. Some of these patients show gall bladder oedema or focal tenderness on ultrasound scanning but in other cases the ultrasound appearances may be entirely normal.

Scintigraphic technique

The technique used is identical with that used for other biliary tract studies already described. It is particularly important to ensure the patients are starved for 4 – 6 hours before the procedure since hepato-biliary agents do not enter the gall bladder in a high proportion of normal patients after eating. Anterior view images of the right upper quadrant are obtained at intervals up to 60 minutes, though the examination may be terminated earlier if the gall bladder, bile ducts and intestine are all demonstrated normally. If there is doubt in distinguishing the gall bladder from adjacent duodenal activity, right anterior oblique or right lateral views are useful.

Interpretation The essential feature of interpretation is that the appearance of activity in the gall bladder excludes mechanical or functional obstruction of the cystic duct and effectively excludes acute cholecystitis. The gall bladder should be visible 15 minutes after injection in about half of normal fasting subjects, and in 90% by 30 minutes after injection. All normal gall bladders should be visualized by 60 minutes after injection.

Failure of the gall bladder to be visualized within 60 minutes may be the result of acute or chronic cholecystitis, biliary tract obstruction, or hepato-cellular disease. In the patient with obstructive jaundice or diffuse liver disease

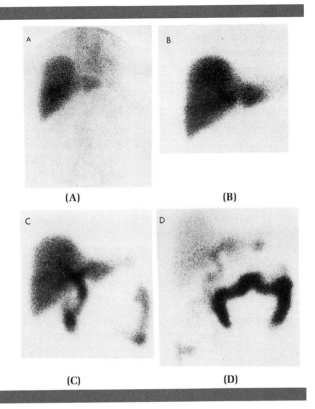

(A)   (B)

(C)   (D)

Fig. 4.8 **Hepato-biliary scintigraphy in acute cholecystitis showing normal uptake in the liver (A, B). Demonstration of the extrahepatic bile ducts and duodenum by 30 minutes after injection (C) but no filling of the gall bladder up to 4 hr after injection (D).**

the excretion of HIDA may be impaired resulting in delay in, or total loss of, visualization of the extrahepatic bile ducts and gall bladder. Where the examination fails to show activity in gall bladder, bile ducts or intestine, the diagnosis of acute cholecystitis cannot be excluded. However, it is still worth carrying out the test in patients with jaundice since the gall bladder will be demonstrated in some cases and cystic duct obstruction can then be excluded.

If activity appears at the expected times after injection in the extrahepatic bile ducts and intestine, but the gall bladder is not visualized the diagnosis of cystic duct obstruction can be made. However, in a small proportion of patients with acute cholecystitis, and a much larger fraction of those with chronic gall bladder disease, activity will appear in the gall bladder between one and four hours after injection (Weissmann et al 1981). Prolonging the examination up to 4 hours allows improved discrimination between acute and chronic cholecystitis (Fig. 4.8 A – D). A scheme of interpretation of HIDA scintigraphy in patients with suspected acute cholecystitis is illustrated in Table 4.1.

Table 4.1 **Interpretation of HIDA scintigraphy in suspected acute cholecystitis**

	Scan pattern	Interpretation
1	Gall bladder demonstrated within 60 minutes of injection	Acute cholecystitis can be excluded
2	Gall bladder not visualized in first 60 minutes despite normal appearance of extra-hepatic bile ducts activity	Gall bladder is diseased, either acute or chronic cholecystitis
3	No gall bladder filling seen up to 4 hours after injection in spite of activity in bile ducts and intestine	Acute cholecystitis extremely likely
4	Gall bladder filling delayed between 1 and 4 hours	Gall bladder disease, probably chronic cholecystitis but possibly acute cholecystitis
5	Delayed or absent visualization of gall bladder, bile ducts and intestine	Obstructive jaundice or diffuse liver disease

Pitfalls in interpretation of HIDA scintigraphy False positive scintigraphic results (ie failure to demonstrate the gall bladder in the absence of gall bladder disease) are occasionally seen in patients with severe intercurrent illness, particularly those on prolonged total parenteral nutrition. Bile stasis is assumed to be the cause; ultrasound scanning often shows echogenic bile within the gall bladder and in some surgical series inspissated viscid bile has been found in the gall bladder at operation. Occasional false negative studies have also been reported in a small proportion of patients with acalculous cholecystitis.

Accuracy of HIDA scintigraphy in acute cholecystitis

Reported figures for the sensitivity and specificity of the procedure vary according to criteria used in interpretation of the images and methods and criteria for verification of the presence or absence of the diagnosis of acute cholecystitis. In several series reviewed by Johnson and Coleman (1982) the overall sensitivity of the test in patients with surgically confirmed disease was between 95 and 100%. In patients in whom the final diagnosis was not acute cholecystitis, the gall bladder was visualized in 76 – 99% (mean specificity 95%). Clearly a normal result has a higher predictive value for absence of disease (close to 100%) than the predictive value of an abnormal result for the presence of disease, but it is in avoiding inappropriate cholecystectomy that the value of the test appears to be greatest.

REFERENCES

Charlton CPJ, Tarlow MJ, Tulley NJ, Harding LK 1988 Biliary atresia: is a 10 minute test useful? Nuclear Medicine Communications **9**: 159

Dick ML, Mowat AP 1986 Biliary scintigraphy with DISIDA. Archives of Diseases in Childhood **61**: 191 – 192

Harding LK, Sorgi M, Wolverson RL, Mosimann F, Sherwin S, Donovan IA et al 1984 The pharmacokinetics of ^{99m}Tc HIDA in man and its relationship to intra-gastric bile acids. Scandinavian Journal of Gastroenterology **19** (Suppl 92): 27 – 29

Harding LK, Donovan IA 1986 Bile dynamics In: Robinson PJ (ed), Nuclear gastroenterology, Churchill Livingstone, Edinburgh pp. 36 – 51

Harding LK, Drumm J, Clarke EA, Donovan IA, Alexander-Williams J 1986 Is gallstone dyspepsia related to duodeno-

gastric reflux? Nuclear Medicine Communications **7**: 281
Johnson AG 1971 Gallstones and flatulent dyspepsia. Cause or coincidence? Postgraduate Medical Journal **47**: 767 – 772

Johnson AG 1972 Pyloric function and gallstone dyspepsia. British Journal of Surgery **59**: 449 – 454

Johnson DG, Coleman RE 1982 New technique in radionuclide imaging of the alimentary system. Radiological Clinics of North America **20**: 635 – 651

Laing FC, Federle MP, Jeffrey RB, Brown TW 1981 Ultrasonic evaluation of patients with right upper quadrant pain. Radiology **140**: 449 – 455

Mosimann F, Sorgi M, Wolverson RL et al 1981 Bile reflux after duodenal ulcer surgery: a study of 114 asymptomatic and symp-tomatic patients. Scandinavian Journal of Gastroenterology **19** (Suppl 92): 224 – 226

Sorgi M, Wolverson RL, Mosimann F, Donovan IA, Alexander-Williams J, Harding LK 1984 Sensitivity and reproducibility of a bile reflux test using ^{99m}Tc HIDA. Scandinavian Journal of Gastroenterology **19** (Suppl 92): 30 – 32

Weissmann HS, Badia J, Sugarman LA, Klinger L, Rosenhatt R, Freeman LM 1981 Spectrum of cholescintigraphic patterns in acute cholecystitis. Radiology **138**: 167 – 175

5 | Liver Disease

INTRODUCTION

Radionuclide imaging was the first non-invasive technique to be widely accepted as a means of demonstrating liver pathology. Its role since the introduction of ultrasonic, CT and MR scanning has evolved to take account of the attributes and advantages of these anatomical methods. This chapter reviews the underlying basis of colloid scintigraphy, the interpretation of normal and abnormal images, the recent development of blood flow studies and other new techniques and the place of scintigraphy in a diagnostic approach to liver disease.

COLLOID SCINTIGRAPHY

Theory The liver colloid scintigram is a map of the distribution of reticuloendothelial (RE) cells within the field of view – normally in liver, spleen, bone marrow and lung. Colloid particles are removed from the circulation by phagocytosis into the RE cells and then remain there. The rate at which colloid is extracted from the blood is closely related to the number of RE cells in the tissue being perfused. Since the mass of the liver in adults is normally eight to ten times that of the spleen, the distribution of intravenously injected colloid is approximately 90% to liver and 10% to spleen – with a small fraction entering bone marrow.

With the number of particles typically used for diagnostic procedures the mechanism for trapping colloid is far from being saturated, so the rate of extraction remains constant at different blood concentrations of colloid. This means that blood clearance and liver uptake can be represented by single exponential curves. The extraction efficiency for normal liver tissue is over 90%, so with liver and spleen together receiving about 25% of the cardiac output, the uptake is rapid with a plasma half-life of 2 – 3 minutes in a healthy individual.

Particle size varies according to the preparation used. Sulphur colloid made by the acid-thiosulphate method has particles ranging from about 30 to 1000 nm in diameter, while most of the commercial freeze-dried colloids have a narrower size range and some have many smaller particles (down to about 3 nm). Larger particles tend to be extracted preferentially by the spleen, whereas with small particles there is a relatively greater uptake into bone marrow.

The size of the smallest lesion detectable by scintigraphy is limited by physical and biological factors. With conventional collimation – inevitably a compromise between count rate efficiency and rejection of scattered radiation to improve spatial accuracy – the resolution of the gamma camera is approximately 8 – 10 mm for a 'cold' lesion. Further degradation in resolution occurs from the superimposition of counts from tissues at different depths and scattering of radiation by overlying soft tissues. Add to this the effects of movement of the patient during acquisition of the image, and the 1 – 2 cm respiratory excursion of the liver and it is not surprising that the technique can detect only lesions of 1 – 2 cm size at the liver surface and larger lesions deep within the liver. Methods for improving the sensitivity of liver scintigraphy for detecting small lesions are discussed further below.

Preparation For static scintigraphy patients require no preparation, but for blood flow studies patients should be fasted for a minimum of four hours in order to avoid the increase in portal flow associated with eating.

Technique and dosimetry The usual administered activity for an adult is 100 – 120 MBq of ^{99m}Tc-sulphur colloid. This gives an absorbed radiation dose of 8 – 12 mGy to the liver and spleen, and a whole-body radiation dose of about 0.5 mGy. Imaging is carried out 15 minutes after injection for patients with normal liver function; in patients with jaundice or known liver impairment a longer delay is desirable. Anterior, posterior, right anterior oblique, right posterior oblique, and both lateral views are obtained. An additional anterior view with lead strips marking the costal margins is also helpful. In the majority of patients the respiratory excursion of the liver is less in the erect than in the supine position, but the difference is only small. In about one-third of patients the amplitude of liver movement when upright is greater than or the same as that when supine. There is, therefore, no great advantage in choosing one or other position to reduce respiratory motion (Harauz & Bronskill 1979).

Interpretation of liver colloid images

Liver size Although it is usual to comment on the size and shape of the liver, these vary so much in the normal population that only major abnormalities can be detected with confidence. Measuring the vertical height of the anterior liver image in the mid-clavicular line (Rosenfield & Schnieder 1974), estimating the area of the anterior image by planimetry (Naftalis & Leevy 1963) and measuring liver volume using a tomographic technique (Grime et al 1983) can all increase the precision of liver size assessment. Whether an accurate knowledge of liver size contributes to improved management of patients with suspected liver disease is yet to be proven. Liver size is more usually assessed subjectively, taking into account the age, build and size of the patient.

Liver shape Attempts have been made to define normal variations in liver shape. Caroli & Bournville (1962) described five normal shapes from a sample of 37 patients; McAfee et al (1965) specified twelve shapes from a sample of 66 normal livers, while Mould (1972) needed 39 varieties to cover a sample of 125 normal livers. The normal liver is pliable enough to vary its shape a little during the respiratory cycle, and moving from the supine to the erect position alters both its shape and its position within the abdomen. An anterior image of the most common liver shape is shown in Figure 5.1. Clearly some varieties of liver shape occur commonly and are easily recognizable as

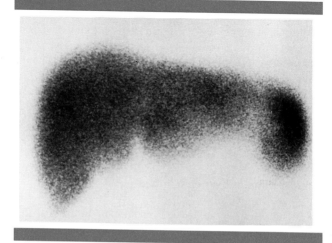

Fig. 5.1 **Normal liver scan.**

normal, but to distinguish the abnormal from the unusual is extremely difficult. Changes in liver shape which occur as a result of pathology are usually accompanied by other indications of abnormality in the images; diagnosing liver disease on the sole basis of abnormal liver shape is fraught with uncertainty. Nevertheless, it is well recognized that relative enlargement of the left lobe occurs in cirrhosis, the caudate lobe is often enlarged in Budd–Chiari syndrome, and mass lesions may cause localized bulges in the liver margins.

Homogeneity Reticuloendothelial cells are distributed uniformly within the liver, and the number of colloid particles injected is enough to produce a uniform distribution of radioactivity within normal liver. Focal liver lesions produce areas of reduced activity in the image; heterogeneous uptake (patchy) is seen with widespread small mass lesions or diffuse parenchymal disease. In either case the scintigraphic appearance probably results from uneven blood flow, with relative ischaemia in the diseased areas, together with replacement of normal liver tissue by tumour or fibrosis.

Colloid shift The uptake of colloid in liver, spleen and bone marrow depends on their blood flow and extraction efficiency. Even in severe liver disease there is only a modest loss of extraction efficiency, so the major mechanism for reduced uptake of colloid is altered blood flow. In diffuse liver disease both intrahepatic and extrahepatic shunting contribute to a reduction in effective liver blood flow. Splenic blood flow is usually increased, and this, together with the reduction in effective liver perfusion, leads to an increase in the proportion of colloid taken up by the spleen.

In the normal subject, counts per unit volume in the liver and spleen are roughly equal, and when measured in a posterior view image liver and spleen uptakes are of about equal density. An increase in the spleen-to-liver ratio is seen in many patients with liver disease, but can also indicate increased splenic blood flow from any other cause. Bone marrow activity, however, is not increased by hypersplenism, and its appearance is a good indicator of diffuse liver disease. Spinal marrow is normally just visible on the posterior view when liver and spleen are correctly exposed; visibility of bone marrow in the anterior view, particularly if ribs are shown, is a strong indication of diffuse liver damage.

Spleen size The spleen varies in size with the size and age of the subject. Methods for estimating splenic size have been described based on linear, planimetric or volumetric measurements. The ability to make a precise measurement does not, however, solve the problem of what is normal, so subjective interpretation of splenic enlargement is still practised. Spleens which are enlarged as a result of portal hypertension show increased colloid uptake, whereas those spleens which are enlarged by infiltration usually show normal or decreased uptake.

Ascites Ascites can often be recognized on images of patients with severe liver disease when the chest wall is outlined by bone marrow uptake and the liver is seen to be displaced medially. Separation between liver and lung activity is also seen in patients with marked ascites.

Lung uptake of colloid The uptake of colloid by lung tissue was initially described as a pre-terminal event in patients with severe liver disease who also had diffuse lung infection, tumour infiltration, or intravascular coagulation. More recently it became apparent that a shift of colloid to the lung occurs in some patients with no recognizable lung pathology; it is still, however, a sign of poor prognosis.

Left-to-right lobe ratio Normally the right lobe of the liver is substantially larger than the left lobe, so that an estimate of their relative colloid uptake would show a R:L ratio of 2 − 3:1. Patients with cirrhosis often show reversal of this ratio because the left lobe is less affected by the pathological process and undergoes compensatory hypertrophy.

Detecting mass lesions by colloid scintigraphy

The scintigraphic appearance of a circumscribed liver lesion is non-specific. Not only tumours but also abscesses, cysts, haematomas and areas of dense fibrosis are devoid of functioning reticuloendothelial cells. Small masses may be obscured by scattered radiation from surrounding liver tissue and lesions close to the surface of the liver may be indistinguishable from impressions or indentations of the liver surface caused by extrahepatic structures. Liver masses must be distinguished from areas of reduced uptake caused by normal anatomical features such as distended hepatic veins in the middle of the superior liver margin, the gall bladder fossa on the inferior margin, indentation on the posterior surface caused by the right kidney, and the lateral indentation caused in some patients by the costal margin. Reduced activity at the porta hepatis is seen in patients with dilated bile ducts, (sometimes the branching structure is clear) or with enlarged lymph nodes in the porta. Areas of diminished activity caused by a pendulous breast or roll of fat around the middle of the patient can usually be recognized and confirmed by obtaining images with the patient supine.

While the appearance of a small number of relatively large lesions is typical for metastases from gastrointestinal tumours, primaries which spread through the systemic circulation more typically produce large numbers of small lesions spread throughout the liver. Liver enlargement is usually a late feature.

Techniques for improving the sensitivity of static scintigrams

Motion correction The respiratory excursion of the liver tends to obscure small lesions and to blur the edges of larger ones. Electronic motion correction has given improved clinical results but during respiration the liver changes not only its position but also its shape, so that the fidelity of the corrected image is better at the centre than the periphery of the liver. Parkin (1980) used a respiratory strain gauge to trigger a multiple-gated acquisition as used with cardiac studies, so producing a sequence of images of the liver obtained at different phases of respiration. The sharpness of clinical images is improved with this method but it requires a prolonged acquisition time.

Image processing Computer processing of images can be used to enhance the conspicuity of abnormalities, usually by means of spatial filters which produce smoothing or edge enhancement effects. Improvements in observer performance, as assessed by ROC curves, have been found when appropriate image filters are applied to simulated lesions in liver phantoms (Houston & Macleod 1979; Cole 1982). However, image filters tend to enhance fluctuations in count density due to normal anatomy as well as those due to pathology and an increase in false positive interpretations may be expected.

Single photon emission tomography (SPET) Volume acquisition using a rotating gamma camera allows axial, sagittal and coronal slices to be obtained. Approximately 10% more liver lesions will be seen on the tomographic images compared with the conventional planar images.

Limitations of this technique include the additional acquisition time required, the degrading effect of respiratory motion, and the great susceptibility of the images to changes in performance characteristics of the gamma camera.

SPET studies allow estimation of liver volume in vivo more accurately than conventional scintigraphy. They also allow measurement of the proportion of the injected dose of colloid taken up by the liver, which correlates well with the clinical and biochemical criteria of severity of disease.

Liver metastases

Significance In the staging of patients with malignant disease the presence of liver metastasis is of major significance. For example, it is clear that the survival of patients with surgically treated colorectal cancer is much more closely linked to the presence of occult liver metastases than to local staging of the primary tumour (Finlay & McArdle 1986). Attempts at curative resection may be considered in patients in whom liver metastases are solitary or limited to a single segment or lobe. The survival of patients following such resections appears to be improved compared with untreated patients with similar solitary or unilobular disease (Adson 1983).

Detection Although used in many studies as the yardstick by which the accuracy of imaging techniques are measured, laparotomy underestimates the incidence of liver metastases. Goligher (1941) in reviewing patients who had undergone surgery for colorectal cancer, found 31 patients who came to autopsy within a month of laparotomy during which the liver had been pronounced normal. Autopsy showed liver metastases in 5 out of these 31 patients (16%). In a post mortem study of 150 livers containing metastases, Ozarda & Pickren (1962) found that in 11% of cases the liver looked and felt normal at its surface but contained deep-seated lesions on sectioning. Finlay et al (1982) described a two year follow-up of patients in whom the liver appeared normal at laparotomy for primary colorectal cancer. Metastases developed in 11 out of 37 such patients (30%). Only six patients had overt metastases at the time of initial surgery, so that the sensitivity of laparotomy compared with two year follow-up was 6 out of 17 cases or about 35%. Since the vast majority of patients with colorectal cancer who die from metastatic disease do so within two years of resection of the primary, it seems likely that their liver deposits are present at the time of surgery. In this context a technique is needed which will detect early liver lesions which cannot be seen or felt by the surgeon. Results with scintigraphic perfusion techniques are encouraging in this respect.

Limitations of imaging techniques The resolution of gamma cameras is such that lesions smaller than 1 – 2 cm at the surface of the liver or 3 – 4 cm if deeply situated, will often be missed. Marginal improvements may be obtained with the use of motion correction devices, image post-processing, and emission tomography. A static liver scintigram with multiple metastases is shown in Figure 5.2.

Lesions in the size range 1 – 2 cm will be more reliably detected by CT, MR and ultrasound than by conventional scintigraphy, but all of these techniques will miss many lesions under a centimetre in size.

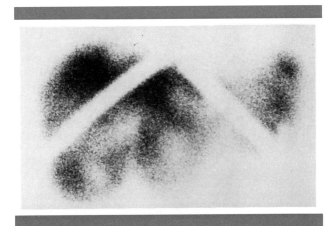

Fig. 5.2 **Anterior view of liver with costal margin markers and showing multiple mass lesions throughout left and right lobes in a patient with colorectal cancer.**

Differential diagnosis of liver masses

Methods of increasing the specificity of liver scintigraphy

A. *Blood flow* With rapid dynamic images, increased flow in the arterial phase is seen with most tumours whether benign or malignant (Fig. 5.3). Cysts and areas of fibrosis

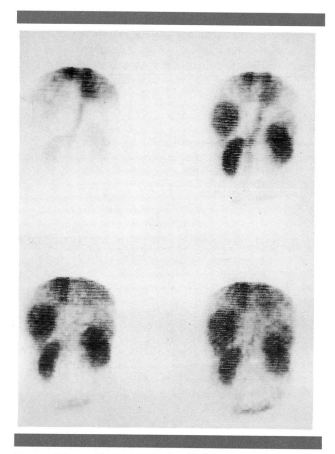

Fig. 5.3 Sequential images of the abdomen during first passage of injected pertechnetate through liver and kidneys in a patient with a hepatocellular carcinoma. Note that flow to the tumour is virtually simultaneous with flow to kidneys indicating arterial supply rather than portal venous inflow.

appear avascular, whereas mature abscesses may show a ring of increased blood flow at the periphery of an otherwise bloodless lesion (DeNardo et al 1974).

B. *Blood Volume* Scintigraphy using intravascular tracers such as ^{99m}Tc-labelled red cells or albumin distinguishes those regions with increased blood volume. Appearances of blood pool images generally parallel those of flow studies with only hepatomas and some benign tumours appearing more active than normal liver whereas cysts, abscesses, metastases, cholangiocarcinomas and areas of fibrosis all appear less active than normal liver. Haemangiomas often produce a disparity between flow and blood volume images since although these lesions may contain large vascular spaces and appear active on blood pool images, the flow through them is usually diminished.

Primary liver tumours

A. *Haemangioma* The most common primary liver tumour, haemangioma, is usually an incidental finding during examination of the liver. Most of these tumours are small, discrete, solitary and produce no clinical symptoms. A minority present clinically with liver enlargement or a local abdominal mass and they may bleed. Symptomatic lesions are treated surgically or by embolization but the usual clinical problem is to differentiate asymptomatic lesions from malignant liver tumours. Biopsy can be avoided if imaging techniques can make a specific diagnosis; this is often possible. Scintigraphic flow studies show reduced perfusion in both arterial and portal phases and the lesions are inactive on both colloid and gallium images. The characteristic feature is the appearance of an area of increased blood volume seen on blood pool images (Front et al 1981, Moinuddin et al 1985). Findings on dynamic CT are also sometimes characteristic, a clear-cut low density lesion close to the surface of the liver showing marked vascular enhancement at its rim during the flow phase with varying degrees of delayed parenchymal enhancement.

B. *Adenoma* Hepatic adenomas when large enough to present clinically are usually inactive on colloid scintigraphy (Welch et al 1985) and show reduced vascularity on flow studies. Active uptake of gallium and of ^{99m}Tc-HIDA has been reported in some cases. Since only liver cells produce bile it has been suggested that scintigraphy with biliary agents such as ^{99m}Tc-labelled HIDA should distinguish between tumours arising in liver cells and other intrahepatic masses. Some intake of ^{99m}Tc-HIDA has been described with hepatic adenomas, focal nodular hyperplasia, and in both primary hepatoma and its metastases.

C. *Focal nodular hyperplasia (FNH)* The scintigraphic features of FNH are variable. Widely but not universally regarded as a tumour, FNH is the one liver lesion in which functioning reticuloendothelial cells are commonly found. On colloid scintigraphy the lesions may be active, inactive or indistinguishable from normal liver. Vascularity is usually increased and uptake of ^{99m}Tc-HIDA is a recognized finding.

D. *Carcinoma* The manifestations of hepatocellular carcinoma are also variable. Most commonly it appears as a solitary mass with increased arterial flow (Fig. 5.3) but in some cases it is multifocal or diffuse and metastatic spread within the liver is common. By the time of diagnosis the tumour has often spread to involve both left and right lobes and the liver is almost always enlarged. Uptake of gallium is seen in about three-quarters of hepatomas but this feature does not correlate well with cell type or alpha-fetoprotein levels (Nagasue 1983). Negative gallium scans are most likely to be seen with avascular or poorly differentiated tumours. Uptake of ^{99m}Tc has been recorded in both primary and secondary hepatoma (Lee & Shapiro 1983).

Cholangiocarcinoma is avascular and inactive on all the scintigraphic techniques mentioned.

E. *Other lesions* Abscesses, cysts and haematomas all appear inactive on colloid HIDA and blood pool scintigraphy but imaging with gallium shows active concentrations at sites of infection in liver abscesses or suppurative hepatitis.

An approach to the diagnosis of focal liver lesions

The superior anatomical resolution of CT, MR and ultrasound when compared with scintigraphy means that the former techniques should be able to detect smaller lesions within the liver. However, in spite of its physical limitations, scintigraphy appears to be approximately as accurate as the anatomical techniques in detecting which patients harbour metastases since most patients have multiple lesions of varying size. When screening is required for large numbers of patients with primary malignancies, the logistic and economic disadvantages of CT and MR may outweigh the marginal advantage of their superior resolution. Ultrasound is relatively cheap and widely available but is much more subjective than scintigraphy and is not as amenable to quality control. Quantitative flow studies have recently been shown to be more sensitive than any other technique in detecting metastases from colorectal cancer; applications in the management of other malignancies are still being studied.

The diagnostic problem of the solitary liver lesion affects a much smaller number of patients so the use of multiple imaging techniques does not impose the same logistic problem as does the screening of large numbers. Cysts and mature abscesses are most easily distinguished from solitary tumours by ultrasound or CT but their avascular nature can be predicted if a liver flow study is carried out; this can be conveniently done as part of a routine scintigraphic examination. The differentiation of solid liver tumours is usually based upon histology, but before carrying out a percutaneous core biopsy it is advisable to check the vascularity of the lesion and for this purpose a scintigraphic flow study is simpler and less invasive than arteriography. Haemangiomas are usually asymptomatic incidental findings and it should be possible to avoid surgical exploration of these patients by a combination of scintigraphy, ultrasound, and CT.

The detection of hepatoma in patients with cirrhosis is often difficult. Sequential scintigraphy showing the development of a focal defect together with liver enlargement is very suggestive but often the colloid images show features of cirrhosis with patchy activity and areas of reduced function. Needle biopsy of the abnormal areas is usually conclusive but biopsy may be undesirable in patients with the coagulation deficiencies of chronic liver disease. In some patients ultrasound, CT and MR show characteristic abnormalities but in others these techniques are also inconclusive. Gallium scintigraphy when combined with colloid imaging allows hepatoma to be distinguished from fibrotic liver in the great majority of cases but is by no means infallible. Unfortunately, those hepatomas which are difficult to detect by scintigraphic methods are usually the ones in which the anatomical techniques are also unsatisfactory and in some of these cases biopsy is also inconclusive. However, most hepatomas will be diagnosed by a combination of scintigraphic and anatomical imaging methods.

Scintigraphic features of diffuse liver disease

Cirrhosis Figure 5.4A shows the typical scintigraphic features of a patient with established cirrhosis – small liver, large active spleen, increased bone marrow uptake, ascites, and heterogeneous liver activity. Patients with cirrhosis secondary to chronic heart failure, amyloidosis or schistosomiasis may have enlarged livers, but in the majority of cases of postnecrotic or alcoholic cirrhosis the liver is normal-sized or small. The right lobe is usually more severely affected than the left so that relative enlargement and increased colloid uptake in the left lobe is seen (Fig. 5.4B). Splenic enlargement is common and increased spleen/liver uptake ratio is often striking. With decreasing liver function, bone marrow uptake increases and in severe cases lung uptake may also be seen (Fig. 5.4C). The distribution of colloid within the liver becomes patchy, sometimes to the extent of mimicking mass lesions; this indicates large areas of fibrosis. Hepatoma developing in a cirrhotic liver poses a diagnostic problem which is considered below.

Hepatitis In acute viral hepatitis the liver appears normal or shows heterogeneous uptake although rarely large filling defects may be seen. The spleen is usually of normal size,

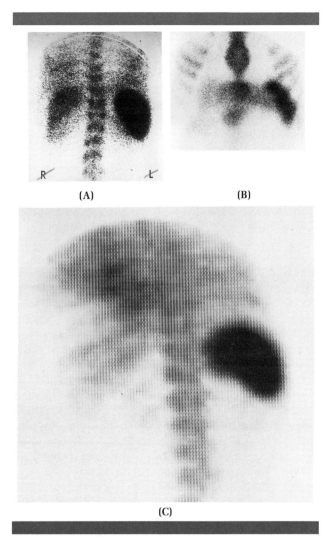

(A)

(B)

(C)

Fig. 5.4 **Colloid images of the upper abdomen in three patients with cirrhosis. A, large active spleen, increased bone marrow uptake and small liver with heterogeneous uptake. B, pronounced uptake in ribs and sternum with small patchy liver showing particular predominance of left lobe uptake. C, hardly any uptake in the liver, very active spleen and bone marrow with also pronounced lung uptake.**

and colloid shift to spleen and bone marrow is not marked. Liver size is usually normal or increased, but with fulminant hepatitis a reduction in liver size is a poor prognostic feature, as is lung uptake of colloid.

In chronic active hepatitis scintigraphy shows patchy liver uptake with colloid shift and often a degree of splenic enlargement but the latter is usually less marked than in cirrhosis. Patients with acute alcoholic hepatitis show similar changes, which can often be reversed by abstinence.

Fatty liver Diffuse fatty infiltration of the liver may produce a normal scintigraphic appearance but usually the liver is enlarged and shows heterogeneous uptake. The spleen size is usually normal and colloid shift is not a prominent feature unless the fatty infiltration is secondary to alcoholic injury.

Amyloid Colloid scintigraphy in hepatic amyloidosis typically shows liver enlargement with patchy activity. Occasionally the images are normal, and rarely large focal lesions are shown. Patients with hepatic or splenic deposits show focal or diffusely increased activity on scintigrams obtained with bone-scanning agents (Fig. 5.5). This is not a recognized feature of other infiltrative liver disorders, although some malignant tumours also show uptake of bone-seeking radionuclides.

Other diffuse liver lesions In granulomatous hepatitis enlargement of both liver and spleen is common, with varying degrees of colloid shift and heterogeneous liver activity (Valdez & Herrera 1968).

Glycogen storage disease typically produces hepatosplenomegaly, with diminished but homogeneous liver uptake of colloid. Focal lesions are sometimes seen and may represent hepatic adenoma or carcinoma, both of which have been associated with this condition (Miller et al 1978).

Liver radiotherapy causes clear-cut areas of reduced or absent function; chemotherapy with anti-tumour agents can produce transient abnormalities including liver enlargement, colloid shift, and heterogeneous uptake (Kaplan et al 1980).

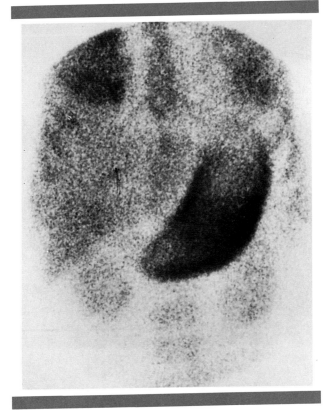

Fig. 5.5 **Bone scintigram – upper abdominal image of a patient with amyloid showing marked increased uptake in the lungs, liver and stomach.**

Reduced but uniform liver uptake with colloid shift is also seen in patients with myelofibrosis, diffuse lymphoma or leukaemic liver infiltration. The same features together with heterogeneous uptake are described in heart failure, obstructive jaundice and diffuse metastatic disease.

Budd–Chiari syndrome This condition presents in young adults with abdominal pain, ascites and liver enlargement. In most cases some or all of the hepatic veins are thrombosed but occasionally venous obstruction results from webs in the cava or hepatic vein ostia, or from tumour invasion. Underlying causes include polycythaemia rubra vera, oestrogen-containing oral contraceptives, hepatoma and trauma, but in many cases no predisposing cause is identified (British Medical Journal 1979, Tavill et al 1975). The characteristic feature seen in many cases of Budd–Chiari syndrome is reduced uptake over the affected liver segment together with locally increased uptake in the caudate lobe seen close to the midline in the anterior view and centrally placed within the liver in the lateral view (Fig. 5.6 A, B). In addition, there is usually a marked reduction in total liver uptake and increased activity in bone marrow, lungs and spleen; the spleen is not usually enlarged except with pre-existing portal hypertension or polycythaemia. Ascites may also be visible on the scan. In some patients with Budd–Chiari syndrome the caudate lobe is not preferentially perfused; scintigraphy then shows the non-specific features of diffuse liver disease.

Definitive diagnosis of Budd–Chiari syndrome requires the histological demonstration of centrilobular necrosis

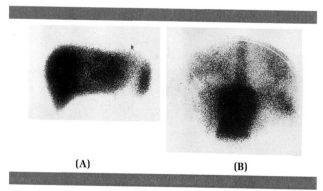

(A) (B)

Fig. 5.6 Colloid images during development of Budd–Chiari syndrome. A, colloid image at initial presentation showing essentially normal appearance. B, colloid image of same patient after onset of acute ascites, portal hypertension and liver decompensation, showing large active caudate lobe, reduced function in the rest of the liver, increased lung and bone marrow uptake with ascites separating the lung and liver margins.

and the typical venographic appearance of spidery collaterals with major vein occlusion. Although ultrasound and CT can show patent hepatic veins, it is less easy to be certain about the absence of patent hepatic veins using these techniques. Since scintigraphy shows characteristic abnormalities in many cases its use should precede biopsy.

The detection of diffuse liver disease

The accuracy of clinical criteria in detecting diffuse liver disease is unknown. Biochemical tests of liver function are occasionally normal in patients with histological and clinical evidence of liver disease, and positive tests occur in some patients with no other evidence of abnormality. Liver biopsy incurs the risk of sampling error, and pathologists do not always agree on interpretation. There is no doubt that scintigraphy is more sensitive than ultrasound or CT scanning in detecting diffuse liver disease (Biello et al 1978, McLees & Gedgaudas-McLees 1984) but it is less sensitive than histology in detecting early liver disease which is truly diffuse. Scintigraphy may be more sensitive than biochemical tests in patients with stable disease, particularly if the lesions are patchy.

Discriminating between different liver disease Studies of the specificity of scintigraphy in distinguishing different liver pathologies almost invariably rely on biopsy histology as the final arbiter. A confident diagnosis by an experienced pathologist will usually be reliable but a significant proportion of biopsies will be insufficiently characteristic for a diagnosis to be reached. For example Baggenstoss (1966) found 25% of 800 biopsies to be indecisive. Most studies of biochemical tests in liver disease rely on biopsy histology for a final diagnosis, so it is not surprising that the limitations of the 'biochemical profile' approach in differentiating liver disorders are similar to those of histology. With 800 biopsies Baggenstoss (1966) was able to reach a correct morphological diagnosis (ie to distinguish cirrhosis, biliary obstruction, hepatitis, fatty infiltration etc) in about three-quarters of his cases. However, the success rate in defining features which indicated the cause of the liver lesion (ie alcoholic versus viral hepatitis, postnecrotic versus biliary cirrhosis) was very substantially less.

A. *Scintigraphic discrimination* The overlap between the range of liver volumes in health and in disease is too great to allow size to be used as a valid discriminator, except in cases of gross hepatomegaly. The patients with the largest livers are likely to have extensive malignancy but their scintigrams almost inevitably show markedly heterogeneous uptake or clear-cut mass lesions. A change in the size of the liver over a period of observation may be more significant. Marked splenomegaly is most likely to be seen in patients with cirrhosis or chronic active hepatitis, much less commonly with fatty infiltration or malignancy. The discovery of lesser degrees of splenomegaly does not aid discrimination.

Marked heterogeneity of liver uptake commonly occurs in malignancy and cirrhosis but is not seen in patients with fatty infiltration or hepatitis uncomplicated by cirrhosis. The latter disorders may however show minor degrees of non-uniformity as do some patients with cholestasis.

A marked colloid shift into the spleen and bone marrow is also seen more commonly in cirrhosis than in other liver lesions. In many patients with alcoholic cirrhosis the right lobe is small while the left lobe is of normal size or enlarged. Measuring the ratio of colloid uptake between the left and right lobes is a sensitive and a specific indicator for alcoholic cirrhosis (Schreiner & Barlai-Kovach 1981). Just as with the biochemical tests a multivariate analysis improves overall discriminations. For example, if colloid shift is marked in relation to the degree of non-uniformity of liver uptake, the probability of cirrhosis is increased; if there is marked heterogeneity with a normal size spleen and relatively little colloid shift then metastases are much more likely. Nevertheless, individual exceptions do occur and minor degrees of abnormality are in general of little discriminatory value. Just as estimates of the sensitivity of scintigraphy in detecting diffuse liver disease (83% by Geslien et al 1976; 93% by Wasnich et al 1979) are of limited practical value since they are based on highly selected groups of patients, attempts to derive predictive values for specific combinations of scintigraphic features are unlikely to be of much clinical use. However, since some patients with stable liver diseases have normal biochemistry and sampling errors with needle biopsy are not inconsiderable, the use of scintigraphy should lead to an overall reduction in uncertainty of diagnosis (Drane & Van Ness 1988). This is particularly apparent in those areas where characteristic scintigraphic patterns are seen in patients whose biochemistry and histology is inconclusive.

LIVER BLOOD FLOW STUDIES

Theory Normal liver receives about 20 – 25% of its blood supply from the hepatic artery and 75 – 80% via the portal vein. Portal venous flow increases physiologically after eating and pathologically in some patients with gross hypersplenism but in virtually all types of liver disease the portal blood flow is reduced. Both primary and secondary liver tumours receive their blood supply very largely from the hepatic arteries. The presence of tumours produces an increase in the arterial contribution to total liver blood flow and this change provides a means for tumour detection using a first-pass technique. The measurement of arterial/portal ratio may also be useful in assessing the severity of liver disease in patients with portal hypertension, and sequential measurements can indicate the progress of disease or the response to treatment.

Many methods for measuring liver blood flow have been developed, but all have disadvantages. Clearance techniques depending upon hepatocyte extraction require hepatic vein catheterization; indicator dilution techniques and electromagnetic flowmeters measure total volumetric flow through the liver and not the effective or nutritive flow which is the clinically significant figure. The ultrasound method is handicapped by non-linear flow and turbulence within the vessels, and postural variations in the cross-sectional area of the portal vein. An ideal technique would measure both total and effective (nutritive) liver perfusion, should be safe, simple, reproducible and non-invasive, and should be effective in the presence of hepatocellular disease (Bradley 1974). The radionuclide methods fulfil some but not all of these requirements. These techniques involve the measurement of the rate of uptake of a bolus of either an absorbable (eg ^{99m}Tc-sulphur colloid) or a non-absorbable (eg ^{99m}Tc-pertechnetate) marker into the liver. This approach does not measure total liver blood flow, but estimates the relative proportion of hepatic arterial to portal venous inflow. This ratio is abnormal both in diffuse liver disease and in hepatic neoplasia.

First-pass techniques Arterial blood reaches the liver directly from the abdominal aorta whereas the portal venous blood first has to traverse the spleen or gut before arriving at the liver. Following an injection of radiographic contrast medium into the the abdominal aorta the hepatic arterial branches are filled within two to three seconds whereas opacification of the portal vein does not begin until after five to fifteen seconds. With the radionuclide techniques the marker is given as a fast bolus injection into a peripheral vein and its arrival at the liver is recorded by a gamma camera and computer. The initial slope of the time/activity curve is proportional to the rate of arrival of tracer within the field of view, so if we can identify separate time periods for the arrival of arterial and portal blood the ratio of the slopes of the time/activity curve during these periods will indicate the relative inflow from the two sources.

Curve analysis and choice of tracer The leading edge of the liver time/activity curve represents hepatic arterial inflow. The estimation of portal inflow is controversial, and several different techniques have been described. Each variation has its own normal range and numerical results obtained with one technique cannot be directly compared with those obtained by a different procedure.

Choosing between an absorbable and a non-absorbable tracer is of major importance. In patients with portal hypertension the colloid technique has several disadvantages: increased extraction of colloid by the spleen reduces the proportion of the injected activity presented to the liver and counting statistics over the liver are correspondingly poor, splenic venous blood dilutes the mesenteric component to a varying degree, and the presence of collaterals disturbs the speed and direction of flow. Better counting statistics can be obtained with a non-absorbable tracer (eg pertechnetate) owing to the smaller radiation dose involved. In patients who are being investigated for metastatic disease the removal of colloid by the spleen is an advantage. Blood flows more quickly through the spleen than through the gut so with the splenic component eliminated, the time separation between the arterial and mesenteric input phases is wider so allowing the two phases to be more clearly distinguished. The colloid technique also has the advantage that conventional static imaging of the liver and spleen can be obtained as part of a single procedure.

Technique Colloid is used in patients with suspected metastatic disease, whereas in patients with diffuse liver disease a non-absorbable tracer is appropriate. A fast intravenous bolus injection of either 120 MBq of ^{99m}Tc-sulphur colloid or 400 – 600 MBq of ^{99m}Tc pertechnetate or ^{99m}Tc diphosphonate is given. The patient, who has starved for at least 4 hours, is positioned supine over a large field of view gamma camera. Image data is acquired as 2-second frames for 60 seconds. From summed images showing the position of lungs, liver, spleen and kidneys, regions of interest are generated for the liver (avoiding the lung bases, right kidney, aorta and vena cava) and for the right kidney. Time/activity curves are generated; the peak of the renal curve is designated Tp. If the bolus is of adequate quality (half rise-time of renal curve eight seconds or less) the average gradient of the liver curve is calculated for two 8-second periods immediately before and after Tp. These are regarded as being proportional to hepatic arterial and portal venous inflow respectively. The ratio of the slopes of these two segments of the curve is the hepatic perfusion index (HPI) (Fig. 5.7).

Applications and results

A. *Colloid tracer – metastatic disease* In normal subjects

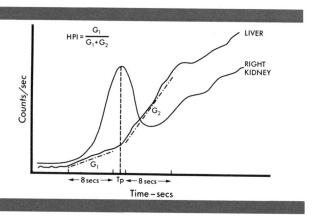

Fig. 5.7 **Stylized time/activity curves from liver and kidney during first pass colloid study. Hepatic perfusion index is calculated as shown from the gradients of the arterial and portal phases of the liver curve.**

the portal phase of the liver curve is much steeper than the arterial phase; this relationship is lost or reversed in patients with liver tumours. In normal subjects HPI averages 0.25 with a range of 0.1 – 0.4. The HPI is elevated in almost all patients with overt liver metastases (Fig. 5.8, Parkin et al 1983). Some patients in whom the liver appears free of disease at laparotomy also have elevation of the HPI. These patients have a high risk of developing metastases within the next two years, whereas patients in whom the HPI is normal have only a low risk (Fig. 5.9, Leveson et al 1985).

B. *Non-absorbable tracer – diffuse liver disease* Figure 5.10 shows the results of pertechnetate flow studies in normal controls and in patients with various types of diffuse liver disease. Flow indices for control subjects ranged from 0.15 to 0.42. Patients with established cirrhosis, portal vein occlusion, surgical portosystemic shunts, and non-cirrhotic diffuse liver disease all had flow indices greater than 0.5. The degree of elevation of HPI correlates fairly well with other indices of severity of liver damage (Bolton et al 1988) and sequential measurements may be useful in monitoring the progress of disease and response to treatment (McLaren et al 1985).

The pathophysiological basis for changes in HPI is not entirely clear. The increased arterial supply to the liver to patients with portal hypertension and in those with large liver tumours is very obvious on X-ray angiography. The subtle changes in patients with early metastatic disease are less easy to explain. In some cases it is clear that the portal component of inflow to the tumour site is virtually abolished, while the arterial component remains or is increased. Experimental data shows that increases in HPI are found within a few days of inoculation of tumour cells

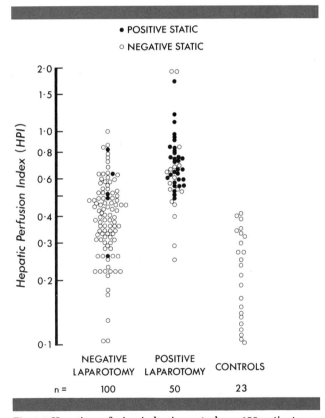

Fig. 5.8 **Hepatic perfusion index in controls on 150 patients with primary gastrointestinal malignancies. 'Positive laparotomy' indicates patients in whom the surgeon was able to see or feel liver metastases at laparotomy.**

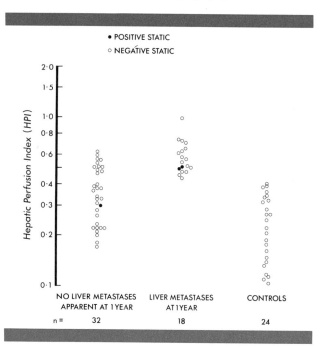

Fig.5.9 Initial pre-operative HPI measurements in 50 patients with no surgical evidence of metastases at the time of resection of the primary tumour. Note strong correlation between initial elevation of HPI and subsequent development of overt metastases.

into the portal vein (Nott et al 1987); this effect is probably caused by arterial/portal shunting rather than physical obliteration of portal radicals by tumour.

Liver microsphere angiography

More direct approaches to liver perfusion scintigraphy have been developed alongside attempts to treat liver tumours by direct local perfusion of chemotherapeutic agents. Hepatic arterial anatomy is very variable with as many as 30 – 40% of subjects having accessory or replaced lobar arteries, so the recognition of ectopic or additional branches to the liver is of major importance if this route is being used for chemotherapy. When accessory or replaced

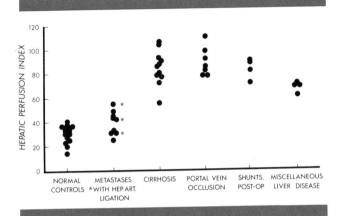

Fig. 5.10 **HPI measurements using non-absorbable tracer in controls and patients with various liver disorders.**

arteries are occluded, perfusion to the affected areas of the liver is rapidly replaced by collateral flow (Koehler et al 1975). If the perfusion catheter is placed so proximally that a substantial fraction of the flow by-passes the liver, drug toxicity is increased (Yang et al 1982). Daly et al (1985) used intra-arterial injection of labelled macroaggregated albumin to assess the vascularity of liver tumours, and were able to predict the likely response to chemotherapy in patients with metastases from colonic cancer. Temporary arteriolar blockade within the liver by biodegradable microspheres may be used to increase the therapeutic response to intra-arterial drugs (Zeissman et al 1983, Mavor et al 1987).

REFERENCES

Adson MA 1983 Hepatic metastases in perspective. American Journal of Roentgenology **140**: 695 – 700

Baggenstoss AH 1966 Morphologic and etiologic diagnoses from hepatic biopsies without clinical data. Medicine **45**: 435 – 443

Biello DR, Levitt RG, Siegel BA, Sagel SS, Stanley RJ 1978 Computed tomography and radionuclide imaging of the liver: a comparative evaluation. Radiology **127**: 159 – 163

Bolton RP, Mairiang EO, Parkin A, Ware F, Robinson P, Losowsky MS 1988 Dynamic liver scanning in cirrhosis. Nuclear Medicine Communications **9**: 235 – 247

Bradley EL 1974 Measurement of hepatic blood flow in man. Surgery **75**: 783 – 789

British Medical Journal Editorial 1979 The Budd-Chiari Syndrome. British Medical Journal **1**: 1302

Caroli J, Bournville B 1962 Valeur diagnostique de la scintillo-graphic hepatique. Archives des Maladies de l'Appareil Digestif **51**: 55 – 82

Cole AZ, Croft BY, Brickley JJ, Antharvedi A 1982 Evaluation of digital image enhancement techniques for liver scintigrams. Physics in Medicine and Biology **27**: 63 – 72

Daly JM, Butler J, Kemeny N et al 1985 Predicting tumour response in patients with colorectal hepatic metastases. Annals of Surgery **202**: 384 – 393

DeNardo GL, Stadalnik RC, DeNardo SJ, Raventos A 1974 Hepatic scintiangiographic patterns. Radiology **111**: 135 – 141

Drane WE, Van Ness MM 1988 Hepatic imaging in diffuse liver disease. Clinical Nuclear Medicine **13**: 182 – 185

Finlay IG, Meek DE, Gray HW, Duncan JG, McArdle CS 1982 Incidence and detection of occult hepatic metastases in colorectal carcinoma. British Medical Journal **2148**: 803 – 805

Finlay IG, McArdle CS 1986 Occult hepatic metastases in colorectal carcinoma. British Journal of Surgery **73**: 732 – 735

Front D, Royal HD, Israel O, Parker JA, Kolodny GM 1981 Scintigraphy of hepatic haemangioma: the value of ^{99m}Tc-labelled red blood cells. Journal of Nuclear Medicine **22**: 684 – 687

Geslien GE, Pinsky SM, Poth RK, Johnson MC 1976 The sensitivity and specificity of ^{99m}Tc-sulphur colloid liver imaging in the diffuse hepatocellular disease. Radiology **118**: 115 – 119

Goligher JC 1941 The operability of carcinoma of the rectum. British Medical Journal **ii**: 393 – 397

Grime JS, Critchley M, Roberts M, Morris AI 1983 Single photon emission tomography in the evaluation of chronic liver disease. Nuclear Medicine Communications **4**: 282 – 289

Harauz G, Bronskill MJ 1979 Comparison of the liver's respiratory motion in the supine and upright positions. Journal of Nuclear Medicine **20**: 733 – 735

Houston AS, Macleod MA 1979 An interpretation of computer assisted image processing and display methods in liver scintigraphy. Physics in Medicine and Biology **24**: 1550 – 1557

Kaplan WD, Drum DE, Lokich JJ 1980 The effect of cancer chemotherapeutic agents on the liver-spleen scan. Journal of Nuclear Medicine **21**: 84 – 87

Koehler RE, Korobkin M, Lewis F 1975 Arteriographic demonstration of collateral arterial supply to the liver after hepatic artery ligation. Radiology **117**: 49 – 54

Lee VW, Shapiro JH 1983 Specific diagnosis of hepatoma using ^{99m}Tc-HIDA and other radionuclides. European Journal of Nuclear Medicine **8**: 191 – 195

Leveson SH, Wiggins PA, Giles GR, Parkin A, Robinson PJ 1985 Deranged liver blood flow patterns in the detection of liver metastases. British Journal of Surgery **72**: 394 – 396

McAfee JG, Ause RG, Wagner HN 1965 Diagnostic value of scintillation scanning of the liver. Archives of Internal Medicine **116**: 95 – 110

McLaren MI, Fleming JS, Walmsley BH, Ackery DM, Taylor I, Karran SI 1985 Dynamic liver scanning in cirrhosis. British Journal of Surgery **72**: 394 – 396

McLees EC, Gedgaudas-McLees RK 1984 Screening for diffuse and focal liver disease: the case for hepatic scintigraphy. Journal of Clinical Ultrasound **12**: 75

Mavor AI, Parkin A, Riley A et al 1987 Initial clinical experience with degradable starch microspheres. Nuclear Medicine Communications **8**: 1011 – 1018

Miller JH, Gates GF, Landing BH, Kogut MD, Roe TF 1978 Scintigraphic abnormalities in glycogen storage disease. Journal of Nuclear Medicine **19**: 354 – 358

Mould RF 1972 An investigation of the variations in normal liver shape. British Journal of Radiology **45**: 586 – 590

Moinuddin M, Allison JR, Montgomery JH, Rockett JF, McMurray JM 1985 Scintigraphic diagnosis of hepatic haemangioma. American Journal of Radiology **145**: 223 – 228

Naftalis J, Leevy CM 1963 Clinical estimation of liver size. American Journal of Digestive Diseases **8**: 236 – 243

Nagasue N 1983 Gallium scanning in the diagnosis of hepatocellular carcinoma: a clinico-pathological study of 45 patients. Clinical Radiology **34**: 139 – 142

Nott DM, Grime JS, Yates J et al 1987 Changes in the hepatic perfusion index during the growth and development of experimental hepatic micrometastases. Nuclear Medicine Communications **8**: 995 – 1000

Ozarda A, Pickren J 1962 The topographic distribution of liver metastases. Its relation to surgical and isotope diagnosis. Journal of Nuclear Medicine **3**: 149 – 152

Parkin A 1980 Improved gamma-camera images of the liver using a physiological gating mechanism. British Journal of Radiology **53**: 900 – 903

Parkin A, Robinson PJ, Baxter P, Leveson S, Wiggins P, Giles GR 1983 Liver perfusion scintigraphy method, normal range and laparotomy correlation in 100 patients. Nuclear Medicine Communications **4**: 395 – 402

Rosenfield AT, Schneider PD 1974 Raid evaluation of hepatic size on radioisotope scan. Journal of Nuclear Medicine **15**: 237 – 240

Schreiner DP, Barlai-Kovach M 1981 Diagnosis of alcoholic cirrhosis with the right-to-left hepatic lobe ratio. Journal of Nuclear Medicine **22**: 116 – 120

Tavill AS, Wood EJ, Krell L, Jones EA, Gregory M, Sherlock S 1975 The Budd–Chiari syndrome: correlation between hepatic scintigraphy and the clinical, radiological and pathological findings in nineteen cases of hepatic venous outflow obstruction. Gastroenterology **68**: 509 – 518

Valdez VA, Herrera NE 1968 Granulomatous hepatitis: spectrum of scintigraphic manifestations. Clinical Nuclear Medicine **3**: 393 – 396

Wasnich M, Warren WD, Fomon JJ 1970 Liver panangiography in the assessment of portal hypertension in liver cirrhosis. Radiographical Clinics of North America **8**: 147 – 167

Welch TJ, Sheedy PF, Johnson CM et al 1985 Focal nodular hyperplasia and hepatic adenoma: comparison of angiography, CT, US and scintigraphy. Radiology **156**: 593 – 595

Yang PJ, Thrall JH, Ensminger WD et al 1982 Perfusion scintigraphy (^{99m}Tc-MAA) during surgery for placement of chemotherapy catheter in hepatic artery. Journal of Nuclear Medicine **23**: 1066 – 1069

Zeissmann HA, Thrall JH, Gyves JW et al 1983 Quantitative hepatic arterial perfusion scintigraphy and starch microspheres in cancer chemotherapy. Journal of Nuclear Medicine **24**: 871 – 875

VITAMIN B12 ABSORPTION

Introduction

Vitamin B12 is required for DNA synthesis and so is essential for cell division. Haemopoietic tissue divides rapidly, and deficiency of vitamin B12 becomes apparent as there is an increased time between cell division and the cells become larger (megaloblastic). Anaemia results, and the white blood cells are hypersegmented. As the disease progresses erythroblasts fail to mature and are destroyed in the marrow so that severe anaemia results.

Role of isotopic test Typical blood appearances are of a macrocytic anaemia with leucopenia and hypersegmented neutrophils. A megaloblastic bone marrow and the low serum level of vitamin B12 confirm the cause of the anaemia.

Deficiency of vitamin B12 may be due to: deficiency of intrinsic factor, diseases of the terminal ileum reducing absorption, dietary deficiency in strict vegetarians (vegans), metabolism of vitamin B12 in the gut by bacteria in blind loops, or rarely by the fish tapeworm (Diphyllobothrium).

A radioactive vitamin B12 absorption test is performed with intrinsic factor to differentiate those patients with deficiency of intrinsic factor from the other causes. Intrinsic factor deficiency is usually due to Addisonian pernicious anaemia, but it may also occur following gastrectomy, or rarely as a result of a congenital deficiency.

Method

Theory Vitamin B12 contains cobalt, and may be labelled by incorporating either ^{57}Co or ^{58}Co into the molecule.

Absorption may then be examined using the Schilling test. It is important to starve the patient before starting the test as the intestinal transport sites for vitamin B12 may become saturated (Merrick 1986). The patient is given 0.5 – 2 μg labelled vitamin B12 by mouth, and 2 hours later an intramuscular injection of 1000 μg hydroxycobalamin. This large dose results in both stable and absorbed radioactive vitamin B12 being excreted in the urine by glomerular filtration, and the amount of labelled vitamin B12 in the urine is proportional to the amount absorbed. Alternatively the patient may be given labelled vitamin B12, and vitamin B12 plus intrinsic factor on separate occasions at least three days apart. This is the conventional Schilling test.

There are two main ways of conducting the test. A popular version of the test is to use two capsules, one containing ^{58}Co vitamin B12 and the other ^{57}Co vitamin B12 bound to intrinsic factor (Dicopac®). This allows the test to be completed in 24 hours, but some argue that exchange may take place between the free and intrinsic factor bound vitamin B12.

Procedure The patient should starve overnight and the test is performed first thing in the morning when the two capsules are given together for the Dicopac® test, or the oral vitamin B12 is given for the conventional Schilling test. At 2 hours the patient is given 1000 μg hydroxycobalamin i.m. and may then eat a light meal. The urine is then collected for 24 hours and the excretion of labelled radioactive vitamin B12 determined by gamma counting.

Results Less than 10% excretion over 24 hours is definitely abnormal. The normal range for the Dicopac® test is 12 – 30% for ^{57}Co (bound to intrinsic factor), and for ^{58}Co, 11 – 28%. In normal subjects the ratio of ^{57}Co to ^{58}Co excretion is 1 (range 0.7 – 1.2). In pernicious anaemia the ratio is greater than 1.8. Reduction of excretion both with and without intrinsic factor indicates malabsorption of vitamin B12 and this may be due to any of the other causes of vitamin deficiency described earlier. It should be remembered however that with severe untreated pernicious anaemia there may be malabsorption, and only after treatment will the typical results found in pernicious anaemia become evident.

Problems with the test The greatest problem arises because of incomplete urine collections so that a malabsorption result may erroneously be inferred. A similar problem arises in patients with renal impairment. In the latter case 48 hour urine collection is recommended. Low results may also be obtained if the patient has gastric stasis, or has in error not been given the inactive i.m. vitamin B12.

Dosimetry The effective dose equivalent from the test is low, 0.2 mSv, and the critical organ is the liver, which receives 3 mGy.

Alternative tests Once vitamin B12 has been established, differentiating Addisonian pernicious anaemia from the other causes requires an absorption test. No other test is reliable: 50% of patients show intrinsic factor antibodies in the serum, and parietal cell antibodies are found in 80%, but may also be found in those without the disease.

BILE ACID MALABSORPTION

Introduction
Conjugated bile acids are reabsorbed in the terminal metre of the ileum. Normally 95% of bile acid is reabsorbed, and circulates 6 to 10 times a day (Merrick 1986). With resection of the terminal ileum malabsorption is inevitable. In other situations bile acid malabsorption may be less evident, and difficult to diagnose.

Role of the nuclear medicine test
Diarrhoea typical of malabsorption is watery, occurs predominantly after meals, and rarely occurs a night. Any steatorrhoea is minor in degree. In addition to being caused by resectional disease of the terminal ileum, it may be idiopathic (including some patients characterized as having irritable bowel syndrome), or associated with vagotomy or

cholecystectomy. This latter post-surgical group may be caused by incompetence of the ileocaecal valve (Merrick 1988), or alternatively surgery may unmask a bile acid transport defect (Fromm & Malavolti 1988). Unfortunately medication to treat bile acid malabsorption is unpalatable, and may require some time to achieve the correct dose. In addition cholestyramine may have an anti-diarrhoeal affect unrelated to its bile sequestrating action, and it is also expensive.

Method

Theory Bile acid malabsorption may be tested using SeHCAT. This is a taurine conjugate of a synthetic bile acid (23 selena 25 homotaurocholate) labelled with ^{75}Se, which is absorbed in the bowel within a short time of oral administration and enters the enterohepatic circulation. It is more resistant to bacterial decay than naturally occurring bile acids and so will give a normal result if there is a bacterial overgrowth in the small intestine, unlike the breath test described later.

SeHCAT is administered orally and the amount retained in the body, typically over a seven-day period, is determined. Normal excretion approximates to the single exponential (Merrick 1986).

Procedure After an overnight fast the patient is given a capsule of SeHCAT (370 KBq). The count rate is recorded using an uncollimated gamma camera positioned over the mid abdomen and as far away as possible from the patient as the room size will allow. Both anterior and posterior views are taken. The geometric mean of these counts at 3 hours represents 100% retention. Retention is measured again at seven days using the same technique. From the technical point of view it is important to include gamma ray energies which extend into the Compton scatter, so that small changes in spatial distribution of the radiopharmaceutical do not affect the result.

Alternatively a whole-body counter may be used when, a smaller amount of SeHCAT (37 KBq) is sufficient.

Results Normally more than 15% of the SeHCAT is retained over seven days. Results less than 8% are definitely indicative of bile acid malabsorption (Merrick 1986). Patients with ileal resection show very low retention values, generally less than 2%. Abnormal results may be obtained in some cases of inflammatory bowel disease affecting the terminal ileum, and sometimes after irradiation of the bowel. In those with results between 8 and 15% there may or may not be a response to cholestyramine.

Problems with the test SeHCAT is expensive and the test tends to overestimate the actual degree of bile acid malabsorption (Fromm & Malavolti 1986).

Dosimetry The effective dose equivalent from 370 KBq of SeHCAT is 0.3 mSv, with the gall bladder being the critical organ receiving 1.2 mGy.

Alternative tests The breath test as described below may be undertaken. Alternatively the patient may be given ^{14}C-labelled taurocholate and its faecal excretion determined. However it is difficult to obtain complete stool collections, and like most tests involving faecal analysis is unpopular with staff and patients. A more recently available test is the bile acid excretion (Merrick 1986) in faecal samples collected over three days.

BREATH TESTS

Introduction
Isotope breath tests have been available to study malabsorption for over 20 years. The specificity and sensitivity of these tests has been criticized, and they have not been used commonly. However the bile acid breath test is helpful to show bile malabsorption or small bowel bacterial overgrowth, and the test using triolein absorption is used in some centres.

Role of the isotopic test

Bile acid absorption Patients with bacterial overgrowth in the small intestine present with steatorrhoea, and may have deficiency of iron, vitamin B12, or folate. The overgrowth results from underlying disease of the small bowel causing stasis, such as a blind loop (afferent loop after gastrectomy or gastroenterostomy), jejunal diverticula, Crohn's disease with stricture formation or ileocolic fistula. Those with bile acid malabsorption present as described in the above section.

Fat absorption Steatorrhoea may be due to a variety of causes, of which bacterial overgrowth is a less common cause. It may occur with pancreatic insufficiency, after gastric surgery, in coeliac disease, extensive Crohn's disease, abdominal lymphoma, or lymphangiectasia of the mesenteric lymphatics.

Methods

Theory The principle of breath tests is straightforward. The patient is given a ^{14}C-labelled compound. At intervals they are asked to breathe into a vial containing a fixed amount of alkali (hyamine) solution until the indicator in the vial changes colour. This shows that a predetermined amount of CO_2 has been liberated in the breath, and the amount of ^{14}C can be determined by liquid scintillation counting in a beta counter. It is then necessary to assume a basal rate of CO_2 production (9 mmol kg^{-1} h^{-1}) in order to express the results as a percentage of the amount of ^{14}C administered.

Procedure

A. *Bile acid absorption* 200 – 400 KBq of ^{14}C-cholyl glycine is administered with a standard meal to the fasting subject. A breath sample is collected as described above every 30 minutes for six hours, and the total amount of ^{14}C determined from the area under the excretion curve.

B. *Fat absorption* The fasting patient is given 200 kBq of ^{14}C-triolein together with a standard meal containing 20 g of fat. Breath is collected over 8 hours as described above and the peak excretion determined.

Results

A. *Bile acid absorption* Normally less than 2% of the administered activity is excreted in the breath over 2 hours (Merrick 1986). Abnormal results arise from two causes. Firstly with intestinal hurry there may be bile acid malabsorption so that the cholyl glycine is broken down in the large bowel. Secondly there may be bacterial overgrowth with the bile acid being deconjugated in the small intestine. In either case the total amount of ^{14}C exceeds 2% of the amount administered (Merrick 1986).

B. *Fat absorption* The lower limit of normal for peak ^{14}C excretion is 3.4% with the normal range of 3.4 − 6.3% of the administered dose (Reba & Salkeld 1982). Impaired fat absorption occurs in steatorrhoea, but not in diarrhoea of other causes. Patients with malabsorption show values of 0 − 3.4% of the administered dose and in some series results correlate with faecal fat determinations, although others have found a poor relationship (Reba & Salkeld 1982).

Problems with the test One of the fundamental assumptions of these tests is that the endogenous CO_2 production is constant. Should this not be the case the sensitivity of the test is reduced. In practice the assumption does not hold with increased metabolic activity (for example due to pyrexia), when pulmonary function is impaired, if the acid base status is upset, or if more than 100 kilocalories is given with the meal as part of the test (King & Toskes 1983).

Generally breath tests tend to be of low sensitivity and specificity. While the bile acid absorption test is regarded as of value it has a false negative rate of 30%. There is much dispute about the value of fat absorption tests (King & Toskes 1983, Reba & Salkeld 1982).

Dosimetry For ^{14}C tests using 200 − 400 KBq of tracer, the typical EDE is 0.1 − 2 mSv. Concerns have been raised about retention of ^{14}C in the fat pool, but these are probably unjustified. The gonad dose is low at 0.1 mGy.

Alternative tests

A. *Bile acid* For bile absorption the other tests are listed above. In the case of bacterial overgrowth, duodenal aspiration and culture has for many years been considered the standard test, although in some patients with positive breath tests several aspirates of the jejunum for coliform and anaerobic organisms have to be made in order to establish the diagnosis.

B. *Fat absorption* Faecal fat excretion is the standard test, although it is not popular with patients or staff.

GASTROINTESTINAL PROTEIN LOSS

Introduction
Excess protein loss from the gastrointestinal tract is a non-specific finding which may occur in many diseases. However it may be useful to determine the exact extent of the protein loss, or alternatively to establish if hypoproteinaemia is due to gastrointestinal protein loss or not.

Role of the isotope test
Conditions in which large amounts of protein are lost include protein-losing enteropathy, infiltration of lymphatics of the colon, severe congestive heart failure, and in some cases of Crohn's disease.

Method

Theory The patient is given $^{51}CrCl_3$ intravenously. Trivalent chromium binds to the serum protein and in particular to transferrin. Normally there is only a small amount of transferrin metabolized each day, and by collection of the stools the amount of protein loss can be calculated.

Procedure Blood is withdrawn into a syringe containing 3 – 4 MBq of $^{51}CrCl_3$ and then reinjected (Merrick 1988), or the isotope may simply be given intravenously. In some departments a blood sample is taken at 10 minutes and the protein loss related to the serum level. Others prefer to relate the faecal counts to a radioactive standard prepared in vitro.

A five-day faecal collection is made and the amount of ^{51}Cr lost is determined.

Results Transferrin metabolism results in up to 2% of the ^{51}Cr being lost in the faeces over the five-day period. Figures above this are abnormal.

Problems As ^{51}Cr is excreted in the urine the main problem with the test is urine contamination of the faeces. Misleading results will, of course be obtained if the faecal collection is incomplete or if the patient suffers from gastrointestinal haemorrhage during the course of the faecal collection. Care must be taken as chromium is absorbed easily onto glass or plastic (Reba & Salkeld 1982).

Dosimetry After administration of $3 - 4$ MBq ^{51}Cr the EDE is 1.7 mSv, and the critical organ the spleen (20 mGy).

Alternative tests The amount of alpha-1-antitrypsin in the stools may be determined and compared with the serum concentrations. This has the advantage of not requiring a radioactive tracer, but is not available in most hospital clinical chemistry departments.

SMALL INTESTINAL AND COLONIC MOTILITY

Introduction
Transit through the gastrointestinal tract depends on four factors: oesophageal transit, gastric emptying, small intestinal transit and colonic transit. Oesophageal transit and gastric emptying are considered in other chapters. Small intestinal and colonic transit are somewhat more difficult to measure.

Role of the isotope test
Altered transit is an important factor in diseases such as irritable bowel syndrome, idiopathic constipation,

ulcerative colitis, and autonomic neuropathy. It has also been used to measure factors affecting drug absorption.

Method

A method of determining small bowel transit of a meal was described by Read et al (1986). For small bowel transit studies they described a meal consisting of mashed potato, baked beans and Frankfurter sausages, with 10 MBq of ^{99m}Tc sulphur colloid incorporated into the mashed potato. As a dessert the patient was given homogenized pineapple in custard, and finally 100 ml of water to drink. Davis et al (1986) have used a light breakfast. Gamma camera images of the abdomen are then taken at 5-minute intervals for the next 8 hours. The stomach is identified on early images and the colon on the later ones. Any other activity is presumed to be in the small bowel. Curves are generated by the computer showing emptying of the stomach, transit through the small bowel, and entry into the colon.

Normal results There is a wide variation of small bowel transit times in normal subjects and the head of the meal takes 2.8 hours (SD±1.5 hour) to reach the colon (Read et al 1986). Mental stress slows transit, pain speeds it up. There is also a variation with the phase of the menstrual cycle, transit being rapid just after menstruation. The mean small bowel transit time was 4 hours (SD±1.4 hour). Colonic filling was complete in 8.6 hours (SD±1.5 hour).

Abnormal results For irritable bowel syndrome, results generally fall in the normal range. However, in patients with diarrhoea, transit times tend to be at the lower end of the normal range. Those presenting with pain and distension tend to have slow small bowel and whole-gut transit.

In chronic constipation there is delayed small bowel transit, and the colon may show colonic inertia or outflow obstruction.

Problems The main problem of the test is overlap between the small bowel and the caecum, and also between the stomach and small bowel. Delineation of the colon may also be difficult.

Alternative tests The alternative test for determining intestinal transit is the breath hydrogen test, which measures stable hydrogen production after a lactulose meal. Breath hydrogen (King & Toskes 1983) is a useful test to determine the arrival of the head of the meal in the colon, where bacteria release hydrogen. However, 20 – 25% of subjects do not have hydrogen-producing bacteria in their colon.

Transit of barium through the bowel is not a very reliable marker of transit, but incorporation of barium into the food by feeding the patient radio-opaque markers at intervals is a satisfactory method of studying whole-bowel transit items.

R E F E R E N C E S

Davis SS, Hardy JG, Fara JW 1986 Transit of pharmaceutical dosage forms through the small intestine. Gut **27**: 886 – 892

Fromm H, Malavolti M 1986 Bile acid induced diarrhoea. Clinics in Gastroenterology **15**: 567 – 582

King CE, Toskes PP 1983 The use of breath tests in the study of malabsorption. Clinics in Gastroenterology **12**: 591 – 610

Read NW, Al-Janabi MN, Holgate AM, Barber DC, Edwards CA 1986 Simultaneous measurement of gastric emptying, small bowel residence and colonic filling of a solid meal by use of a gamma camera. Gut **27**: 300 – 308

Reba RC, Salkeld J 1982 In vitro studies of malabsorption and other gastrointestinal disorders. Seminars in Nuclear Medicine **12**: 147 – 155

Merrick MV 1986 Assessment of the small intestine. In: Robinson PJ (ed) Nuclear gastroenterology. Churchill Livingstone, Edinburgh pp. 157 – 169

Merrick MV 1988 Small intestine. In: Rhys Davies E, Thomas WEG (eds), Nuclear medicine: applications to surgery. Castle House Publications, Tunbridge Wells, pp. 62 – 74

Meckel's Diverticulum

CLINICAL CONSIDERATIONS

Autopsy studies reveal the presence of a Meckel's diverticulum in 1 – 2% of the population. The proportion of patients in whom the diverticulum causes symptoms is disputed but is probably less than 20% (Mackey & Dineen 1983); they may present at any age, most commonly in the first decade of life. Symptoms are believed to arise from peptic ulceration within the diverticulum causing local pain, bleeding or scarring leading to local inflammation or small gut obstruction. Ectopic gastric mucosa is found only in a minority of asymptomatic Meckel's diverticula but is found in most of the cases which present clinically.

Scintigraphic detection of Meckel's diverticulum depends upon the localization of injected pertechnetate within ectopic gastric mucosa contained in the diverticulum. The technique is simple, requires only a single intravenous injection, takes under an hour to perform, and carries a very low radiation burden. The reliability and accuracy of the test vary in different reports but in a large multi-centre series (Conway 1980) the procedure correctly identified the presence or absence of a Meckel's diverticulum in about three-quarters of patients who subsequently underwent surgery. This compares favourably with the small bowel barium technique of enteroclysis and with arteriography, both of which can show the presence of Meckel's diverticula in a substantial proportion of cases, but both of which also impart a greater radiation burden and are essentially more invasive procedures.

Although the incidence of symptomatic Meckel's diverticula in clinical practice is low, the non-invasive nature of the scintigraphic test makes it appropriate to use for screening patients with unexplained gastrointestinal bleeding and normal upper tract endoscopy, and also in patients with unexplained abdominal pain and normal endoscopy, particularly children in whom the pain is episodic.

Technique

Theory When pertechnetate is injected intravenously it diffuses into the extracellular fluid space but is also selectively cleared from the circulation by the thyroid, the salivary glands, the choroid plexus of the brain, and the gastric mucosa. The mechanism for the concentration of pertechnetate in the gastric mucosa is not entirely clear. The rate of clearance is such that maximum uptake is achieved in most adult patients between 15 and 30 minutes after injection, and after a shorter time in children. In addition to being concentrated within the gastric mucosa, pertechnetate is also secreted into the lumen of the gut and will then be free to move along to adjacent segments of bowel. The prior administration of H2 blocking agents reduces or abolishes the secretion of pertechnetate into the lumen in the majority of patients.

This test visualizes gastric mucosa both in the stomach and in ectopic sites, eg Meckel's diverticulum, oesophagus, duplication cysts.

Radiopharmaceutical The agent used is sodium pertechnetate containing 100 – 200 MBq of ^{99m}Tc.

Preparation The patient should starve overnight to ensure that the stomach is empty and to reduce the rate of secretion of gastric juices. With infants and small children it is enough to withhold one feed. H2 blockade using cimetidine (or equivalent preparations) is recommended. The adult dose is 600 mg given on the evening before the test and 400 mg on the morning of the test. Doses for children should be scaled down according to body surface area.

Acquisition After injection the patient is positioned supine with the gamma camera over the abdomen and pelvis. In the case of infants and small children it is more convenient to lie the patient prone on the surface of the camera.

Images are obtained at five-minute intervals up to 45 minutes after injection. Since pertechnetate is excreted largely through the kidney it is important at this stage to empty the bladder and obtain a further image of the pelvis. Oblique or lateral views of the lower abdomen and pelvis may also be helpful.

Normal appearances The concentration of activity in the stomach normally increases up to 15 – 30 minutes after injection and then remains constant. Renal activity appears early and excreted pertechnetate gradually accumulates in the bladder (Fig. 7.1). Even with the use of H2 blockade, a small proportion of patients will secrete pertechnetate into the lumen of the stomach. Subsequent peristalsis then transfers the activity to the proximal small bowel. Confusion should be avoided by reviewing the time of arrival of activity in the suspected area. The uptake in a Meckel's diverticulum should be synchronous with the accumulation in the normal gastric mucosa. Activity in the ureters may be confusing at first but should be recognized by its transient nature. Oblique or lateral views will also help to distinguish ureteric activity, which is relatively posterior in position, from activity in a Meckel's diverticulum which is relatively anterior.

Technical variations
Pentagastrin may be administered in order to increase the rate of uptake of pertechnetate into the gastric mucosa but it does also have the effect of increasing the rate of secretion into the lumen. An alternative approach has been to inject glucagon simultaneously with the pertechnetate; this inhibits gastric and intestinal peristalsis, so preventing the onward movement of secreted activity. However, glucagon also reduces the rate of uptake of pertechnetate into the stomach. On balance these agents are not recommended.

Abnormal results An area of uptake of pertechnetate which is remote from, but synchronous with, the normal gastric mucosa is suggestive of a Meckel's diverticulum. Most commonly this will be in the right iliac fossa (Fig. 7.2) but it can be almost anywhere in the abdomen. Positive results

93

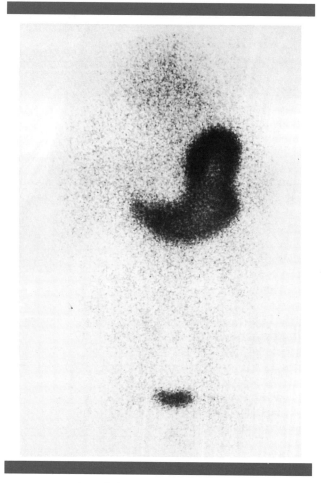

Fig. 7.1 **Normal Meckel's scan. The gastric mucosa is distinctly outlined by pertechnetate; because of renal excretion there is also some activity in the bladder.**

are also seen with other pathologies involving ectopic gastric mucosa, eg duplication cysts. Negative results are obtained in patients in whom the Meckel's diverticulum does not contain gastric mucosa.

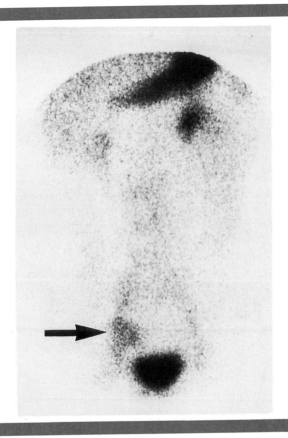

Fig. 7.2 **Pertechnetate scintigraphy in a patient with a bleeding Meckel's diverticulum. In addition to the normal gastric uptake, activity is visible in both kidneys and the bladder but a further focus is seen in the right iliac fossa (arrow).**

REFERENCES

Conway JJ 1980 Radionuclide diagnosis of Meckel's diverticulum. Gastrointestinal Radiology **5**: 209 – 213.
Mackey WC, Dineen P 1983 A fifty year experience with Meckel's diverticulum. Surgery, Gynaecology & Obstetrics **156**: 56 – 64

INTRODUCTION

Tumours of the gastrointestinal tract are common and in the United Kingdom count for 7% of all deaths. Detection at an early stage is difficult. Many of the symptoms such as dyspepsia, weight loss and diarrhoea are non-specific, and imaging tests generally rely on the physical size of the tumour disrupting normal anatomy. In the stomach and colon where endoscopy is easy smaller tumours may be detected. In the past ^{67}Ga (see Chapter 9) was used for detection of gastrointestinal tract tumours, but its sensitivity proved to be very low. Radioimmunoscintigraphy relies on the production of anti-tumour antibodies which are labelled with a radioactive marker. Unfortunately there are no totally specific tumour markers yet available and cross reactivity occurs with different types of tumour and with normal tissues. Recent advances have been made in tumour imaging because of improved antibodies, better radio-labels, and improved imaging techniques.

Role of scintigraphy

Radioimmunoscintigraphy offers the potential of imaging tumours only a few millimetres in diameter. At present however it is generally restricted to staging cases of proven cancer, or in localizing its recurrence in patients with rising carcino-embryonic antigen (CEA) levels in the blood. It is also used to assess the value of anti-cancer chemotherapy.

Carcinoma of the colon is the commonest of the gastrointestinal tract malignant tumours, and radioimmunoscintigraphy may be useful in this situation. Results with the other gastrointestinal tract tumours, such as the stomach and pancreas, have been less successful.

Method

Theory To prepare the antibody mice are injected with an antigen, the spleen removed, and the splenic lymphocytes fused with mouse myeloma cells to form hybrid cells. The cell population is screened to find those which produce the best antibody and these cells are then grown in vitro or in mouse ascites to produce large quantities of the IgG antibody. Protein digestion techniques may then be used to remove the constant part of the antibody molecule (Fig. 8.1) which tends to result in non-specific binding to various

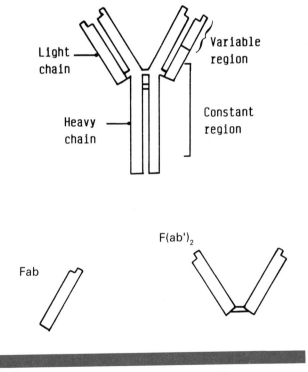

Light chain

Variable region

Heavy chain

Constant region

$F(ab')_2$

Fab

Fig. 8.1 **Structure of an antibody. Removal of the constant region by protein digestion may leave Fab or $F(ab')_2$ fragments.**

body tissues. The resulting Fab or F(ab')$_2$ antibody fragment will then generally show better tumour accumulation.

Such antibodies are prepared to tumour markers expressed by cancer cells. While CEA is most commonly used several antibodies to other antigens expressed by gastrointestinal tract tumours are available (Perkins 1989). CEA is released by a number of types of tumour including those of the colon, stomach, and pancreas. However there may be marked differences in tumour detection rates of anti-CEA antibodies for colorectal cancers despite similar tumour to non-tumour uptake in resected specimens (Perkins et al 1989).

The patient's perception Uptake of antibodies tends to be low, 0.1% per gram with a good antibody (Britton & Granowska 1988) and imaging times may be long. In addition it is usual to take the images at various times after injection of the antibody. However, the technique is non-invasive, and the patient merely has to lie still for imaging.

Because a mouse protein is being injected, patients with atopy or a strong history of allergy to foreign proteins should be excluded. An intradermal skin test with the antibody used to be standard practice, but this is now generally not used since repeated injections of protein result in the loss of tumour uptake as the patient produces antibodies to the mouse protein (Perkins 1989). In any case the value of the skin test in detecting the rare individual who will respond unfavourably to the antibody is doubtful.

Radiopharmaceutical Monoclonal antibodies may be labelled with a variety of radionuclides (Britton & Granowska 1988). ^{131}I has been used for many years and while it has the advantage that the labelling procedure is relatively straightforward, the disadvantages are high radiation dose, poor imaging characteristics, urinary excretion, and uptake of free iodide by the gastric mucosa and the thyroid. The latter problem also exists with ^{123}I, although its imaging characteristics are much better. ^{111}In has been used for a number of antibodies but it is expensive, and there is uptake in the liver and spleen which may confuse interpretation. Recently it has become possible to label antibodies with ^{99m}Tc, but there is liver uptake which limits its use for small liver metastases.

With earlier antibodies, particularly those labelled with ^{131}I, non-specific activity in the blood pool and tissue fluid created confusion in interpreting the images, and it was usual to subtract the image of ^{99m}Tc-labelled albumin and free pertechnetate from that of the antibody. In other words an attempt was being made to subtract the non-specific activity. Subtraction techniques however tend to produce artefacts and if there is sufficient tumour accumulation they are not necessary.

Acquisition Many techniques are used and with different radionuclides the detailed protocol varies. The antibody is injected intravenously and images taken on two or three occasions up to seven days with ^{131}I, 72 hours with ^{111}In, 24 hours with ^{123}I, and 18 hours with ^{99m}Tc (Perkins 1989). Additionally tomography may be required, but recent experience suggests that this is not necessary if there is sufficient tumour uptake of the antibody (Granowska et al 1989). Even so it may be useful, for example, in separating the posterior pelvis from bone marrow activity posteriorly or bladder anteriorly.

A second radiopharmaceutical may be used to image the liver and spleen, or kidneys, in order to permit accurate localization of the site of secondary deposits. Where there is normally liver and spleen uptake of the antibody this may be sufficient for localization.

Normal appearances In theory there should be no uptake of antibodies in the normal subject. However when iodine-labelled antibodies are used urinary excretion occurs, and physiological uptake may be evident in the stomach despite administration of iodide and perchlorate. Uptake in the reticuloendothelial system may be found with ^{111}In or ^{99m}Tc. There may also be bowel uptake but this can generally be differentiated from tumour if it changes in position with subsequent images, or when the patient is given an enema.

Abnormal appearances Examples of abnormal uptake are shown in Figures 8.2 – 8.4.

Dosimetry Typical effective dose equivalent figures (Perkins 1989) of antibodies labelled with 80 MBq of ^{131}I, ^{123}I, and ^{111}In are 10, 6, 10 mSv respectively. Using 400 MBq ^{99m}Tc the corresponding figure is 4 mSv. Radiation doses to individual organs, especially the liver are high: with iodine the absorbed liver dose is 20 – 60 mGy, with [123]I 20 mGy, [111]In 70 – 100 mGy and [99m]Tc 10 – 20 mGy. However, it must be remembered that these agents are used in patients with proven tumours.

Sensitivity Odavic et al (1989) have reviewed the sensitivity of radioimmunoscintigraphy in colon carcinoma; in 11 published series reported between 1980 and 1988 the sensitivity was between 41 and 93%. Recent figures using newer antibodies (Table 8.1) show both a high sensitivity and specificity.

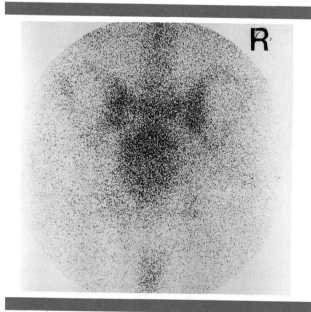

Fig. 8.2 **Posterior images of the upper abdomen and pelvis 72 hr post injection in a patient with a large recurrent rectal tumour. Anti-CEA antibody labelled with** [111]**In. (Courtesy Dr A Perkins, Nottingham.)**

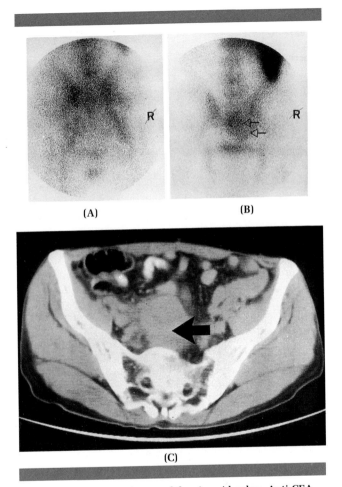

Fig. 8.3 **Recurrent carcinoma of the sigmoid colon. Anti-CEA antibody labelled with ¹¹¹In. A, Posterior blood pool image, showing activity in the great vessels and bone marrow. B, Tumour uptake (arrows) in images at 48 hr. C, Corresponding CT scan. (Courtesy Dr A Perkins, Nottingham.)**

Such results are promising but the experience in many depart-ments is disappointing, probably due to the exact antibody used, lack of experience in interpreting the images, and the types of patients being referred.

101

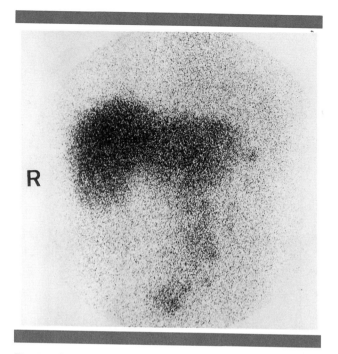

Fig. 8.4 **Anterior images of recurrent stomach cancer, imaged 48 hr after injection. F(ab')2 antibody labelled with ¹¹¹In. Marked uptake in para-aortic lymph nodes. (Courtesy Dr A Perkins, Nottingham.)**

Choice of scintigraphic technique Radioimmunoscintigraphy is used in proven cases of cancer and is particularly valuable with small tumours (less than 2 cm in diameter) which are difficult to detect using other imaging techniques. Mariani (1989) has shown in 70 patients that the sensitivity of radioimmunoscintigraphy is 93% compared with 69% for ultrasound, but it shows no difference compared with computerized tomography. Gasparini et al (1989) on the other hand has shown sensitivities of 92%, 90%, 69% and 36% for NMR, immunoscintigraphy, computerized tomography and ultrasound respectively in 48 patients with suspected local recurrence of colorectal cancer.

While these results are encouraging it must be remembered that the radioisotope technique is time

Table 8.1 **Sensitivity and specificity (%) of radioimmunoscintigraphy in detecting colorectal cancer.**

	Sensitivity	Specificity	No. of patients
Baum et al (1989)	73	88	40
Gasparini et al (1989)	90	–	48
Leinsinger et al (1989)	93	85	80
Mariani et al (1989)	79	97	542

consuming, and if repeated leads to anti-mouse antibodies being formed by the patient. Such tests are of particular value however in detecting small metastases, and in situations where scar tissue or inflammatory change makes the detection of secondary deposit difficult.

REFERENCES

Baum RP, Hertel A, Lorenz M, Hottenrott C, Schwarz A, Maul FD, and Hor G 1989 Tc-99m labelled intact monoclonal anti-CEA antibody for successful localization of tumour recurrences. Nuclear Medicine **(Suppl 25)**: 515 – 518

Britton KE, Granowska M 1988 Radioimmunoscintigraphy In: Rhys Davies E, Thomas WEG (eds), Nuclear Medicine – applications to surgery. Castle House Publications, Tunbridge Wells pp. 300 – 311

Gasparini MD, Crippa F, Regalia E, Seregni E, Bomgardieri E, Buraggi GL 1989 Role of immunoscintigraphy in local recurrences of colo-rectal carcinoma: comparison with other diagnostic methods Nuclear Medicine **(Suppl 25)**: 519 – 522

Granowska M, Richman P, Britton KE, et al 1989 A new monoclonal antibody for radioimmunoscintigraphy of colorectal cancer: PR1A3 labelled with Indium-111. Nuclear Medicine **(Suppl 25)**: 531 – 534

Leinsinger G, Scheidhauer K, Denecke H, Kragh P, Abenhardt A, Moser E, Kirsch CM 1989 Significance of immunoscintigraphy using SPECT and 131-I labeled monoclonal antibodies to CEA/CA-19-9 in the follow-up of colorectal cancer. Nuclear Medicine **(Suppl 25)**: 523 – 526

Mariani G, Rosa C and Donato L 1989 Comparison of the diagnostic sensitivity of tumour radioimmunoscintigraphy by means of an anti-CEA monoclonal antibody with other non-invasive diagnostic techniques. Nuclear Medicine **(Suppl 25)**: 527 – 530

Odavic M, Elakovic M, Djuknic M, Jankovic Z, Rastovac M, Bojanic N 1989 Diagnostic and prognostic reliability of the radioimmunoscintigraphy (RIS) in colorectal carcinoma. Nuclear Medicine **(Suppl 25)**: 535 – 538

Perkins AC 1989 Tumour Imaging In: Sharp PF, Gemmell HG, Smith FW (eds), Practical Nuclear Medicine, IRL Press, Oxford, pp. 287 – 298

Perkins AC, Ballantyne KC, Fromm MV 1989 The clinical role of immunoscintigraphy in gastrointestinal cancer In: Chatal JF (ed), Monoclonal antibodies in immunoscintigraphy. CRC Press, Florida (in press)

INTRODUCTION

Acute infections in the gastrointestinal tract are common, and are generally diagnosed easily and resolve quickly. However, there are three instances of inflammation where diagnosis may be difficult and where nuclear medicine tests are useful. These are inflammatory bowel disease, post-operative sepsis and pyrexia of undetermined origin (PUO).

Inflammatory bowel disease

Inflammatory bowel disease comprises mainly Crohn's disease and ulcerative colitis. Ulcerative colitis is generally easier to diagnose because it predominantly affects the colon which is accessible to sigmoidoscopy and rectal biopsy. Crohn's disease may affect the small bowel only when it produces less clear-cut symptoms. Straight X-ray of the abdomen may show obstruction or a mass in the right iliac fossa. However, the typical changes are usually seen on barium follow-through examinations with mucosal thickening, ulcers, and ultimately stenosis and proximal dilatation. In patients where the colon is involved the diagnosis may be obtained by colonoscopy and biopsy.

Leucocytes migrate to areas of inflammation and infection, and in inflammatory bowel disease they move through the bowel lumen and are excreted in the faeces. Radiolabelled leucocytes are useful both in establishing the presence of inflammatory bowel disease and in assessing its activity, particularly in acute disease or when abscess or fistula are suspected (Becker et al 1988).

In inflammatory bowel disease a combination of conventional blood and radiological tests may miss extensive disease (Elliott et al 1982). Radiolabelled leucocytes have been validated both against clinical indices and histological criteria of inflammation (Saverymuttu et al 1986). There is also a strong correlation of radiolabelled leucocyte excretion with disease activity.

Post-operative sepsis

Abscess formation is a not uncommon complication of abdominal surgical procedures. The presence of the abscess is often evident from the clinical condition of the patient, and the white blood cell count. However, localization of the abscess is required prior to drainage. This is generally achieved using ultrasound, although computerized tomography may at times be helpful when it is available. Even with these imaging techniques some abscesses are difficult to localize, and recurrent abscesses after treatment may give a misleading appearance. Furthermore, pus in the subphrenic and perinephric spaces is generally detected easily, but in the paracolic gutters and in the pelvis diagnostic problems may arise. In addition the patient with operation scars, surgical drains or stoma bags may be difficult to examine with ultrasound and the early abscess cavities without liquefaction may not be detected. In such circumstances radiolabelled leucocytes or ^{67}Ga are used for localization of the abscess. However, because ^{67}Ga is excreted via the colon radiolabelled leucocytes should, whenever they are available, be used when pus in the abdomen is suspected.

PUO

PUO is defined as a fever which persists for three or more weeks and for which no cause is evident. Such cases are usually due to a common condition with an unusual presentation. Tumours are not generally detected using radiolabelled leucocytes unless there is an associated inflammatory response, but some of the tumours which commonly cause PUO, mainly lymphomas, leukaemias and hypernephromas may often show gallium uptake. Of the chronic infections tuberculosis remains a relatively common cause of PUO and this is generally detected better with gallium than with radiolabelled granulocytes, presumably because the inflammatory response is mainly lymphocytic. However, with more acute conditions such as abscess, radiolabelled leucocytes are recommended. In addition certain other causes of PUO may be detected using gallium, for example sarcoidosis. It is important to remember that gallium is a useful agent for localizing an abnormal area, but it is non-specific and the exact nature of the disease must generally be determined by aspiration or biopsy. Sometimes, when the site of the disease is known, it is possible to find the pathological cause on reviewing radiographs or repeating an ultrasound examination.

RADIOLABELLED LEUCOCYTES

Labelling of granulocytes was described over ten years ago and has now been successfully used in many departments. Granulocytes have a half-life in the circulation of 7 hours, and because they migrate to areas of infection are useful for localizing inflammation.

[111]In-labelled leucocytes

Theory ^{111}In is chelated to the white blood cells using tropolone, oxine or other lipophilic agents. Usually mixed leucocytes are labelled but it is possible to label pure granulocytes for specific purposes. Some skill is required in preparing the radiopharmaceutical, and no department should undertake the test without training in a department which has established the technique (Buxton-Thomas 1986).

Radiopharmaceutical Separation of white blood cells from a 30 – 50 ml blood sample takes about one hour, and the remainder of the labelling procedure a further hour, after which time the radiolabelled leucocytes are reinjected. A large gauge needle (gauge 19) is desirable to prevent damaging the white blood cells on reinjection, although in those with poor veins a smaller cannula may be used if the injection is given slowly. In the smaller department ^{111}In may take two working days to obtain, and it costs approximately £60 a vial. In the larger department ^{111}In is a stock order, and up to five labellings could be performed in the same day with one ^{111}In vial.

Acquisition Images are taken after 4 hours in cases of

inflammatory bowel disease, and 24 hours if an abscess is suspected. Some authors have argued that a granulocyte rather than a mixed cell label is important in inflammatory bowel disease, and that the tropolone labelling method is required (Saverymuttu et al 1983). This is not the authors' experience.

Normal appearances Normal visualization of the liver, spleen and bone marrow is evident. Because of the high activity in the spleen and to a lesser extent in the liver, abscesses in these organs may be difficult to detect.

Abnormal appearances Examples of an abscess and acute pancreatitis are shown in Figs. 9.1 and 9.2.

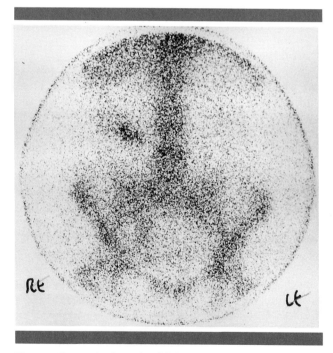

Fig. 9.1 **Abscess in the right abdomen demonstrated using** [111]**In leucocytes. This abscess had remained undetected at two previous laparotomies.**

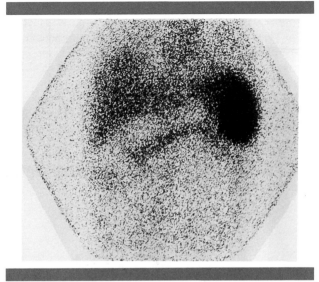

Fig. 9.2 **Uptake in the region of the pancreas using ¹¹¹In leucocytes in a case of acute pancreatitis.**

⁹⁹ᵐTc hexamethyl-propylene amine oxime (HMPAO) leucocytes

Theory This alternative technique has become available in the last two years. It provides images which are improved compared with those obtained with ¹¹¹In because of better imaging characteristics, and a higher affinity of the lipophilic HMPAO for neutrophils. However biliary excretion may confuse interpretation of abdominal images.

A smaller volume of blood, 25 – 30 ml, can be used for labelling, but the need to reinject the cells through a large gauge needle remains. While the cell separation takes the same time as the ¹¹¹In method, the labelling procedure is shorter so that the total labelling time is one and a half hours. There is no day-to-day problem of availability since HMPAO kits may be stored, but the current cost of the radiopharmaceutical is just under £100 per patient, which may prevent more generalized use of this technique.

Inflammatory Disease: Radiolabelled leucocytes

Acquisition Because ^{99m}Tc has a shorter half-life than ^{111}In, the optimal imaging time is earlier using HMPAO-labelled leucocytes. Images are obtained after 1 hour in patients with inflammatory bowel disease, and after 4 hours if an abscess is suspected, although later pictures may be taken.

Appearances There is more bone marrow uptake of HMPAO than ^{111}In leucocytes, some renal excretion, and in later images hepatobiliary excretion (Fig. 9.3) may confuse interpretation of activity in the abdomen.

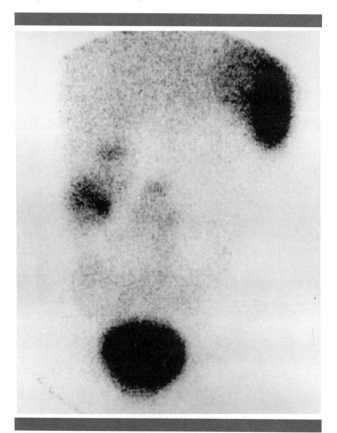

Fig. 9.3 **HMPAO-labelled leucocytes demonstrating an abscess in the right abdomen. There is some diffuse activity due to biliary excretion. (Courtesy of Dr MWJ Hayward, Cardiff)**

Dosimetry of radiolabelled leucocytes The amount of
^{111}In administered by different departments is variable, but
with an administered activity of 10 MBq the EDE is 6 mSv
and the radiation dose to the spleen 72 mSv. This high
dose to the spleen has caused concern, particularly in the
case of children. Using 200 MBq of ^{99m}Tc HMPAO white
blood cells the corresponding EDE is 3 mSv, and the splenic
dose 31 mSv.

Sensitivity In inflammatory bowel disease (Fig. 9.4 A, B)
labelled leucocytes allow discrimination of active and
inactive bowel segments with a sensitivity of 96% and a
specificity of 97%. Abscesses are detected with a sensitivity
of 95% and a specificity of 99% (Becker et al 1988). Positive
images are obtained in other conditions where there is an
inflammatory response such as recent infarcts, and with
some tumours. In addition care has to be taken in
interpreting the images because localized infection due for
example to drip or catheter sites, and surgical scars will be
evident. An accessory spleen is uncommon but may be

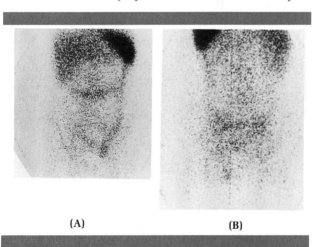

(A)   **(B)**

Fig. 9.4 **A, Image at 4 hr in a case of Crohn's colitis showing
that the disease affects the transverse and descending colon. B,
By 24 hr the leucocytes have moved along the bowel and a
non-diagnostic appearance is obtained (the vertical line is a
film artefact).**

mistaken for an abscess. False positive studies occur with any form of enteritis or colitis and gastrointestinal bleeding may be mistaken for inflammatory bowel disease or abscess. False negative studies occur in patients on steroids, effective antibiotic therapy or immunosuppression, and sometimes with longstanding abscesses where the activity is avascular and walled off. Swallowed leucocytes from infection in the upper respiratory tract have also been described to cause confusion in interpreting abdominal images.

Faecal excretion of ^{111}In leucocytes

Saverymuttu et al (1986) have shown a strong correlation between histological grading of inflammatory bowel disease and faecal leucocyte excretion. They suggest that faecal excretion should be the standard of disease activity in inflammatory bowel disease as long as a granulocyte, rather than a mixed leucocyte, label is used. Over a four-day period the normal excretion is up to 2% of the injected amount of ^{111}In. HMPAO-labelled cells cannot be used for this purpose because of biliary excretion of the radiopharmaceutical. Problems may arise with the test however because of incomplete faecal collection, and in the case of poor leucocyte labelling a falsely high value may be obtained. Finally it must be remembered that this test is popular neither with patients nor nuclear medicine department staff.

^{67}GALLIUM CITRATE

Although first described as a tumour imaging agent, ^{67}Ga has been used for detection of infection since 1971. The mechanism of gallium uptake is poorly understood, but it is carried on proteins, notably lactoferrin, which is bound at sites of infection, and in addition there is uptake of gallium both by leucocytes and bacterial cells.

Radiopharmaceutical Gallium is injected intravenously as the citrate, and no preparation in the hospital radiopharmacy is required. However it generally has to be ordered specially and may take up to 72 hours to be obtained from the manufacturers.

Acquisition For suspected abscess images are taken at 24 hours, although some authors recommend imaging as early as 4 hours. The patient should be given a mild laxative on the day of injection and daily until the test is complete. No other preparation is necessary. 100 – 120 MBq ⁶⁷Ga citrate is injected, and imaging may continue up to 72 hours if a tumour is suspected. Anterior and posterior chest and abdominal films should be taken.

Normal appearances The bone marrow, liver and spleen are normally visualized. The main problem with gallium imaging is excretion of gallium into the bowel (Fig. 9.5). Should there be confusion as to whether activity is in faeces or represents a localized abscess an enema should be given. Should movement of the activity occur its faecal nature is confirmed, but often no change in distribution occurs even if the activity is faecal.

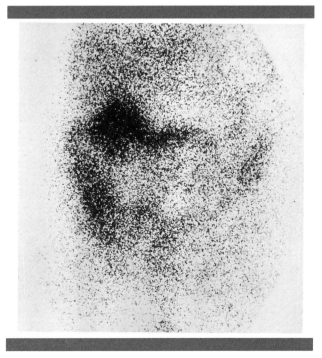

Fig. 9.5 **Gallium images at 24 hr showing an abscess in the upper abdomen but with overlying activity in the colon.**

Abnormal appearances The general criterion of abnormality is comparison with the liver: any uptake greater than that of the liver is considered abnormal. Normal excretion of gallium also occurs into the nasopharynx, and breast uptake is not uncommon. This is more marked in patients taking oestrogens or related drugs such as antiemetics, and especially so in those who have been breast feeding recently. The kidneys may show gallium accumulation in the first 24 hours, but uptake at 48 hours is rare.

Unlike ^{111}In leucocytes gallium will show some longstanding abscesses which exhibit a chronic inflammatory response. As with radiolabelled leucocytes, negative results may be obtained with patients on antibiotics or steroids, but in the case of gallium this may also occur in patients depleted of iron.

Sensitivity Because of the physical characteristics of ^{67}Ga and considerations of dosimetry, images are of poor quality compared with ^{111}In or ^{99m}Tc HMPAO-labelled leucocytes.

A summary of the results from 271 patients included in five publications describing the use of gallium in post-operative sepsis and PUO has been published by O'Mara (1983). The overall sensitivity and specificity was 91%. However, gallium uptake was non-specific. While a high (>80%) proportion of lymphomas take up gallium, the figure is less for hypernephromas (70%) and with the common adenocarcinomas of the gastrointestinal tract only approximately 20% of tumours can be expected to take up gallium.

Dosimetry The 78 hour half-life of gallium is useful in that images can be taken over several days, but results in a relatively high radiation dose with an EDE of 9 mSv for administered activity of only 80 MBq.

REFERENCES
Becker W, Fischbach W, Weppler M, Mosl B, Jacoby G, Barnes W 1988 Radiolabelled granulocytes in inflammatory bowel disease: diagnostic possibilities and clinical

indications, Nuclear Medicine Communications **9**: 693 – 701

Buxton-Thomas W 1986 Radiolabelled white cells in inflammatory disease. In: Robinson PJA (ed) Nuclear Gastroenterology, Churchill Livingstone, New York pp. 116 – 126

Elliott PR, Lennard-Jones JF, Bartram CI, Swarbrick ET, Williams GB, Dawson AM et al 1982 Colonoscopic diagnosis of minimal change colitis in barium enema. Lancet **ii**: 650 – 651

O'Mara RE 1983 Localisation of infection In: Maisey NM, Britton KE, Gilday DL (eds), Clinical Nuclear Medicine, Chapman and Hall, London pp. 391 – 404

Saverymuttu SH, Camilleri M, Rees H, Lavender JP, Hodgson HJF, Chadwick US 1986 [111]Indium granulocyte scanning in the assessment of disease extent and activity in inflammatory bowel disease. Gastroenterology **90**: 1121 – 1128

Saverymuttu SH, Crofton ME, Peters AM, Lavender JP 1983 Indium 111 tropolonate leucocyte scanning in the detection of intra-abdominal abscesses. Clinical Radiology **34**: 593 – 596

INTRODUCTION

For most of the last 2000 years physicians have believed that gastrointestinal bleeding was caused by overloading of the body with blood. Treatment consisted of assisting nature by removing yet more blood; the practice of applying leeches as part of the management of gastrointestinal bleeding died out only about the turn of the present century. More recent experience has indicated that knowledge of the source of bleeding in a patient presenting with haematemesis or melaena is an important factor contributing to improved prognosis, particularly in older people in whom the morbidity and mortality from gastrointestinal bleeding was substantially higher when the bleeding point is not found.

THE ROLE OF SCINTIGRAPHY IN GI BLEEDING

Most patients presenting with haematemesis or melaena will have a source of bleeding found by endoscopy or barium examination. However, in a minority of cases the initial investigations will be negative or inconclusive and it is in this group that scintigraphy has its major role. A positive result will confirm that bleeding is continuing and will direct the angiographer (or the surgeon) to the likely bleeding site. Negative scintigraphy will indicate that the bleeding has stopped so eliminating the requirement for emergency arteriography. Arteriography may still be required to look for a structural vascular abnormality, but this procedure can then be carried out electively. Scintigraphy may also have a supplementary role where endoscopy is relatively contra-indicated (eg shortly after gastric surgery or in patients with hepatitis-associated antigen) and where endoscopic findings are inconclusive (eg colon filled with blood, lesion not seen; or a lesion seen endoscopically but without stigmata of recent bleeding). In patients in whom the source of bleeding has been recognized by the initial procedures, scintigraphy may be used to demonstrate whether or not the bleeding has stopped.

The colloid technique, if positive, gives a rapid and fairly precise localization of the site of bleeding. Intermittent bleeding may be missed by this method so a negative result can usefully be followed up immediately by a labelled red cell test. The techniques are non-invasive and fairly simple to carry out. Since the patients concerned need urgent investigation, it is essential to have an acute on-call service for these procedures to be clinically effective.

Colloid technique

Theory Labelled colloid is rapidly cleared from the circulation by the liver, spleen and bone marrow. If there is active gastrointestinal bleeding at the time of injection, a small radioactive haematoma will appear at the bleeding site. With the blood radioactivity rapidly declining, the haematoma will become increasingly visible through the background within a few minutes. The rate of clearance of labelled colloid from the circulation in the normal human subject is such that the blood half-life is in the region of two minutes. This method therefore depends upon bleeding taking place within a few minutes of the injection. Intense uptake in the liver and spleen may overlie bleeding points in the stomach, duodenum and colonic flexures, so bleeding from these sites will sometimes be detected only on delayed films obtained when the extravasated blood has moved along the bowel.

Radiopharmaceutical Any of the commercially available colloids or an in-house preparation of sulphur colloid can be used, labelled with technetium. The choice of colloid depends upon availability, a major limiting factor being the time taken in preparation. A high binding efficiency is obtained with in-house sulphur colloid preparations but the method takes about an hour to perform, which is an unacceptable constraint for the acutely bleeding patient.

Freeze-dried tin colloid can be labelled within a few minutes and if used immediately should have a high binding efficiency with only a small proportion of unbound pertechnetate. The material needs to be freshly prepared in order to minimize the proportion of free pertechnetate included, as urinary excretion may confuse interpretation of the abdominal images. The activity administered is substantially more than is used for conventional liver/spleen scintigraphy, up to 400 MBq being given.

Acquisition The labelled colloid is given intravenously as a fast bolus. The patient is positioned supine with a gamma camera over the abdomen. A rapid sequence of images (eg nine images at 2 seconds each) is obtained during the first passage of the bolus through the arterial circulation, in order to show abdominal aneurysms and other vascular abnormalities. Subsequently, static images are obtained after 2 and 5 minutes and then at 5-minute intervals up to 45 minutes. After the 2-minute images it helps to mask off the relatively intense activity within the liver and spleen using strips of lead rubber in order to enhance the visibility of any abnormal uptake in the abdomen or pelvis. Oblique views are occasionally helpful to provide another view of the colonic flexures and also to help distinguish large bowel from small bowel locations of extravasated activity. If the patient has a bowel action during the procedure it is important to check the stool for radioactivity; if positive this will not only confirm active bleeding but should facilitate interpretation of the images obtained before and after the melaena was passed.

Normal appearances Blood pool activity outlines the vessels at two minutes but there is already quite marked uptake in the liver and spleen at this stage (Fig. 10.1 A, B). From five minutes onwards the bone marrow, spine and pelvis are increasingly visible and blood background activity becomes progressively less. About half an hour after injection there is often a little accumulation of free pertechnetate in the bladder but this is not a source of confusion since the time sequence of the appearance of bladder activity is quite different from that of intraluminal bleeding. Renal transplants usually take up enough colloid

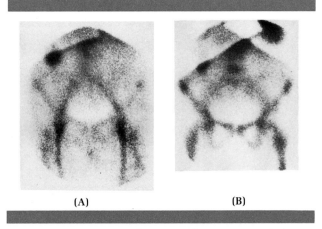

(A)   (B)

Fig. 10.1 **Colloid scintigraphy – normal appearances. A, 2
minutes after injection; B, 10 minutes after injection. Liver and
spleen are partly masked by lead rubber; activity is seen in the
vessels then subsequently in the bone marrow.**

to outline the kidney parenchyma (Fig. 10.2) but marked
uptake is an abnormal feature which has been used as an
indicator of rejection.

Abnormal results Extravasated blood in the intestine is
usually seen within the first few minutes after injection.
Gastric or duodenal bleeding may be masked by the liver,
so extravasation appearing first in the jejunum after 20 –
30 minutes should be taken as an indication of a more
proximal bleeding site (Fig. 10.3 A, B). Extravasated blood
tends to move along the bowel quite briskly so that
sequential images generally show a change in the position
of the abnormal focus. This can be useful in determining
the anatomical site of bleeding. Extravasated activity which
seems to move about fairly quickly in the abdomen is in
the small bowel, that which stays stationary or moves
slowly is probably in the large bowel (Figs. 10.4 A, B, 10.5
A, B). Blood in the colon may occasionally reflux from the
sigmoid back towards the caecum and cases of reflux from
the caecum into the small bowel have been described.

Dosimetry The average adult of 70 kg body weight injected

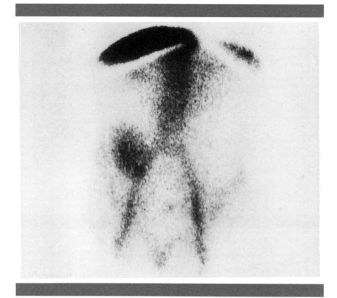

Fig. 10.2 Normal colloid scintigraphy in renal transplant patient showing intake in the kidney approximately equal to spinal marrow uptake.

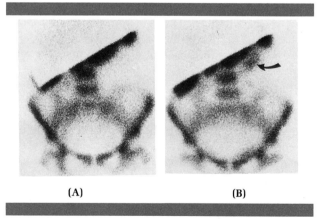

(A)   (B)

Fig. 10.3 Colloid scintigraphy in duodenal bleeding. A, 5 minute image showing normal appearance; B, 15 minute image showing activity appearing for the first time in left upper quadrant (arrow). Duodenal origin subsequently confirmed.

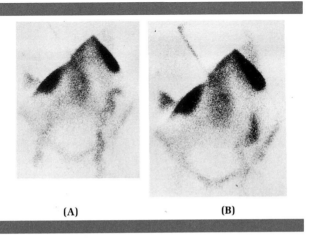

(A)   (B)

Fig. 10.4 **A, B, Images at 5 and 10 minutes after injection in patient with bleeding from diverticular disease in the descending colon.**

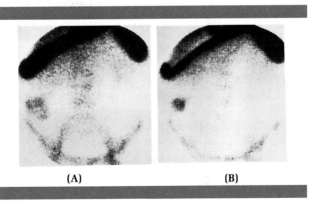

(A)   (B)

Fig. 10.5 **A, B 10 minute images showing stasis of extravasated blood in the right iliac fossa; caecal bleeding site confirmed at surgery.**

with 400 MBq technetium-labelled colloid would sustain an effective dose equivalent of about 6 mSv.

Red cell technique

Theory Autologous red cells labelled with technetium stay in the circulation and with good labelling technique the distribution of intravascular pertechnetate can be followed for up to 24 hours. Extravasation of labelled cells at a bleeding point will produce a radioactive haematoma at the site of bleeding and this will eventually be detectable by the gamma camera. Probably about 70 ml of blood are required to produce a visible 'hot spot' within the bowel by this method, approximately the same volume that is required to produce a melaena stool. However, the successful demonstration of a gastrointestinal bleeding point by this method depends not only upon the rate of bleeding but also upon the rate at which the extravasated blood moves along the bowel lumen and the vascularity of the surrounding structures. This technique is less sensitive than the colloid method in respect of the amount of extravasated blood required before a positive result can be obtained, but has the advantage that the stability of the label within the vascular compartment allows the detection of intermittent or very slow bleeding over a period of several hours.

Radiopharmaceutical Autologous red cells can be labelled with technetium either in vivo or in vitro. In vitro method requires that the red cells are separated from a 10 ml blood sample and incubated with a reducing agent, usually a stannous salt, and subsequently pertechnetate. After incubation the cells are washed and then re-injected into the patient. A simpler in vivo technique can be achieved by first injecting stannous salt intravenously and then a few minutes later withdrawing 10 ml of blood into a syringe containing ^{99m}Tc pertechnetate with a little heparinized saline, allowing the blood to mix in the syringe for several minutes and then re-injecting it back into the patient.

A higher level of binding efficiency and stability is achieved by the in vitro method but this does require a little additional time and expertise.

Acquisition An intravenous injection of up to 400 MBq of technetium-labelled red cells is given as a fast bolus. Anterior view images of the abdomen and pelvis are obtained starting with a rapid sequence of dynamic images during the first pass phase (eg nine frames at 2-second intervals). Subsequent images are obtained at 2 minutes and then at 5-minute intervals up to 30 minutes, at 45 and at 60 minutes. If no abnormality is shown so far, further images are obtained at intervals up to 24 hours.

Normal appearances Initially, vascularity of the liver, spleen and kidneys is sufficient to outline these organs clearly in addition to the cardiac blood pool and major vessels. The small bowel often shows a persistent vascular blush, and in many cases the portal vein is discernible (Fig. 10.6). The appearances change little after initial re-

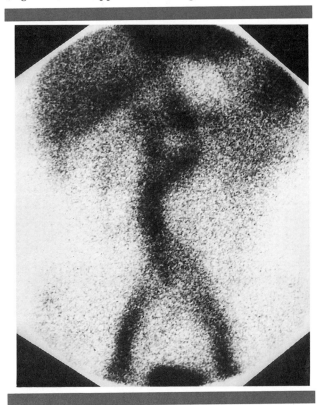

Fig. 10.6 **Abdominal image 60 minutes after injection of labelled red cells showing activity in vascular spaces, liver, spleen and kidneys but no intestinal extravasation (normal appearance).**

distribution of the labelled cells within the circulation but a degree of renal excretion of unbound pertechnetate is quite common, particularly if an in vivo labelling technique has been used.

Abnormal patterns Abnormality is recognized as a focus of radioactivity outside the normal vascular and visceral landmarks, which increases in intensity compared with blood background activity. Sequential images which show a change in position of the abnormal focus help to locate the bleeding point. Blood in the small bowel lumen tends to move along quite briskly producing a fairly rapid change on sequential images while blood in the colon tends to move more slowly along the margins of the abdomen. Extravasation which is first seen on late images in the caecum could indicate a bleeding point in the right colon but might also result from slow or intermittent extravasation from a more proximal site in the small bowel. However, in most cases of small bowel bleeding the distal ileum would be visualized as well as the caecum (Fig. 10.7).

Dosimetry In an average adult of 70 kg body weight injected with 400 MBq of technetium-labelled red cells the effective dose equivalent is 3 mSv.

Sensitivity of the scintigraphic methods

In small experimental animals Alavi et al (1977) detected extravasation into the intestine at rates as low as 0.1 ml per minute using labelled colloid. Although this figure cannot be directly extrapolated to the clinical situation, experimental comparisons between the bleeding rates required for detection by scintigraphy and arteriography show that the colloid method is more sensitive. Using technetium-labelled red cells, Smith & Arteburn (1980) were able to visualize as little as 5 ml of blood introduced into the stomach of a volunteer although other workers have suggested that a larger extravasated volume is required for a positive result by this method. Clearly the sensitivity of either method in clinical application will not achieve the optimum results obtained experimentally, but either test should be sufficiently sensitive to detect gastrointestinal

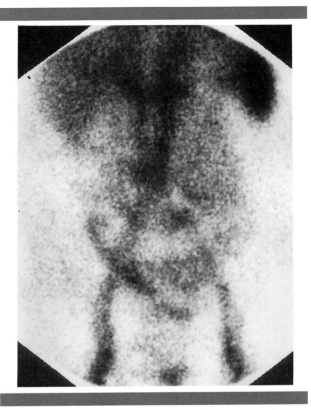

Fig. 10.7 **Abdominal image three hours after injection of labelled red cells showing activity in major vessels, liver, spleen and kidneys but also in several loops of small bowel indicating upper intestinal or gastric bleeding site.**

bleeding of the rate which is sufficient to produce clinically overt melaena. Bleeding which is so slow as to produce only occult blood loss, ie a positive Benzidene or Guiaic test for blood in the faeces, will not be demonstrable by the scintigraphic methods.

The measurement of occult bleeding
If there is a clinical requirement to estimate the rate of gastrointestinal blood loss in patients with slow or occult

bleeding, this can be achieved by labelling a sample of the patient's red cells with up to 4 MBq of ^{51}Cr, which has a half-life of 28 days. After reinjecting the labelled autologous cells, blood samples are taken at 10 minutes and at the end of a period of several days during which all stools are collected. By comparing the radioactivity in the stool collection with that in the two blood samples the volume of blood in the stool can be calculated.

Choice of scintigraphic technique

With the colloid procedure, background radioactivity clears quickly so extravasated blood is seen within a few minutes, as long as it is not obscured by the liver or spleen. With such an early positive result the extravasated blood is shown at or close to the bleeding point so that a confident localization can usually be made at this stage. Activity in the liver and spleen tends to obscure bleeding sites in the stomach and duodenum but an abnormality first seen in the upper abdomen on delayed images will indicate a more proximal bleeding site, and in any case most of these lesions will be detected endoscopically.

Gastrointestinal bleeding is quite often intermittent, and if the patient has stopped bleeding at the time of the colloid procedure a bleeding point will not be shown. A major advantage of the red cell technique is that, since the labelled cells remain in the circulation, intermittent bleeding will eventually produce a positive result as long as repeated observations are made (McKusick et al 1981). However, with a late positive result it is less easy to determine the site of origin of the bleeding than with an early positive colloid result.

A comprehensive approach uses both techniques: first, labelled colloid is given and an early positive result indicates an active bleeding site; if the colloid procedure is negative, red cell labelling can then be carried out and continuing observations made up to 24 hours.

Correlation with arteriography

The bleeding rate at which arteriography will show extravasation of contrast medium is about 0.5 ml per minute in experimental studies, probably double this rate in clinical practice. The time during which the bleeding point is exposed to contrast medium during arteriography is only a few seconds, considerably shorter than the time spent within the circulation by labelled colloid. Venous bleeding is much less easily detected than arterial bleeding by angiography, whereas with the scintigraphic methods the type of vessel involved makes no difference to the result. These reasons explain why, in comparative series, angiography is less sensitive than scintigraphy in detecting the presence of bleeding (Alavi & Ring 1981). In a substantial percentage of cases, positive scintigraphy has been followed by negative arteriography but the reverse has been reported only extremely rarely. Scintigraphy may be used as a screening procedure to select patients for urgent arteriography. Those in whom the scintigraphy is negative are extremely unlikely to have a bleeding point shown angiographically, whereas if scintigraphy is positive the probable site of bleeding can be indicated to the angiographer and the possibility of therapeutic embolization considered.

If scintigraphy is negative, angiography may still be indicated to look for a vascular malformation or similar abnormality even in the absence of active bleeding; this however can be an elective procedure carried out under optimum conditions rather than an emergency investigation.

Clinical correlations

As a general rule, decisions about the replacement of blood loss by transfusion and the requirement for emergency surgery to control bleeding will be based on clinical and haematological findings rather than on the results of imaging. However, it is interesting to note that in studies where scintigraphic results have been correlated with outcome, patients with positive scintigraphy have higher transfusion requirements, a greater probability of rebleeding, are more likely to undergo surgery and stay longer in hospital than those patients in whom scintigraphy is negative.

REFERENCES

Alavi A, Dann RW, Baum S, Biery DN 1977 Scintigraphic

detection of acute gastrointestinal bleeding. Radiology **124**: 753 – 756

Alavi A, Ring EJ 1981 Localization of gastrointestinal bleeding; superiority of ^{99m}Tc sulphur colloid compared with angiography. American Journal of Roentgenology **137**: 741 – 748

McKusick KA, Froelich J, Callahan RJ, Winzelberg GG, Strauss HW 1981 ^{99m}Tc red cells for detection of gastrointestinal bleeding. American Journal of Radiology **137**: 1113 – 1118

Smith RK, Arteburn JG 1980 Detection and localization of gastrointestinal bleeding using ^{99m}Tc-pyrophosphate in in vivo labelled red blood cells. Clinical Nuclear Medicine **5**: 55 – 60

INTRODUCTION

In most circumstances the spleen is imaged using a colloid. However it is sometimes necessary to visualize the spleen alone, and in those circumstances the role of the spleen in removing damaged red cells from the circulation is utilized.

Techniques

Colloid scintigraphy The technique for performing colloid scintigraphy of the spleen is virtually identical with that already described for the liver (see Chapter 5). When examination of the spleen is of prime concern, left anterior oblique and left posterior oblique views should be obtained in addition to anterior, posterior and left lateral images.

Denatured red cells When a demonstration of the spleen completely free of overlapping liver tissue is required (eg in measuring the volume of a small or atrophic spleen) scintigraphy using denatured red cells is required. Red cells are normally sequestered by the spleen and when damaged either by heat or chemical insult the cells are cleared much more rapidly into the spleen. Prior labelling of the damaged cells then allows splenic imaging with very little interference from overlapping liver or other tissues. Although chemical methods for denaturing red cells are well established, the preferred option is to use heat treatment, which is simple to perform and requires no special equipment.

The red cells from 20 ml autologous blood are separated and labelled with approximately 50 MBq of sodium pertechnetate using a standard technique (Dacie & Lewis 1975). The labelled cells are then incubated for 20 minutes at 50°C then reinjected intravenously into the patient.

Static scintigraphic views are obtained 2 hours after injection. Acquisition of images onto computer allows subsequent volume calculation (Roberts et al 1976). The effective dose equivalent is 2 mSv.

Applications

The size of the spleen Clinical examination is insensitive to minor degrees of splenic enlargement and the assessment of more considerable splenomegaly is imprecise and subjective. Imaging methods allow an objective and reproducible estimation of splenic size with considerable accuracy. Parameters described include the maximum bipolar length of the spleen and its surface area in the left lateral view, but the most precise correlation with the weights of subsequently excised spleens is obtained by a volume measurement calculated from anterior, posterior and left lateral views (Roberts et al 1976). The vast majority of adult spleens fall within the size range of 150 – 300 ml although some apparently healthy individuals have spleens which fall outside this range. There is a fairly loose correlation between body size and spleen size, a tendency for the adult spleen gradually to shrink with increasing age, and a small sex difference in that men generally have larger spleens than women.

The breadth of the normal range means that more precise knowledge of splenic volume may not answer the question of whether a particular individual's spleen is enlarged or not, but a baseline measurement does permit a much more precise assessment of changes in spleen size observed subsequently.

Mass lesions in the left upper quadrant Exploration of the anatomy in the left upper quadrant is usually carried out initially by ultrasound or CT scanning. In some cases involvement of the spleen is difficult to define and scintigraphy may be the optimum method for showing whether the spleen is invaded, enlarged or displaced (and if so in which direction).

Anomalies Demonstration of the site of multiple masses of splenic tissue may be the key to the diagnosis of the polysplenia syndrome (bilateral left-sidedness) and the absence of splenic tissue is characteristic of asplenia (bilateral right-sidedness). In both conditions the liver is usually centrally placed and the stomach may be on either side.

Accessory spleens, which may appear on ultrasound or CT to be indistinguishable from other soft tissue nodules in the upper abdomen, can be recognized readily by their uptake of colloid or denatured red cells (Fig. 11.1). The recognition of accessory spleens may be important after therapeutic splenectomy in lymphoma and haematologic disorders, such as idiopathic thrombocytopenia purpura. The preservation of functioning splenic tissue after splenectomy for trauma can be most effectively documented by scintigraphy (Fig. 11.2).

The enlarged spleen Splenic scintigraphy can be used to discriminate the three major types of splenomegaly.

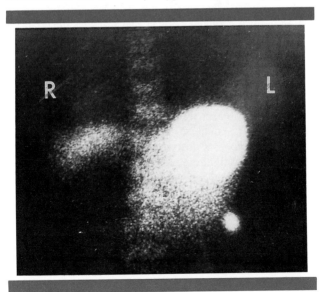

Fig. 11.1 **Accessory spleen at the lower border of the liver visualized by colloid scintigraphy in a patient with severe liver disease.**

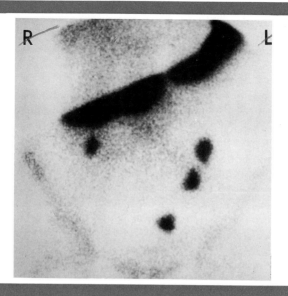

Fig. 11.2 **Anterior colloid image of abdomen after splenectomy for trauma. During the operative procedure small slices of spleen were impacted in the omentum in order to preserve a degree of splenic function.**

(a) Hypersplenism implies enlargement of the spleen without abnormal tissue being present. This category includes patients with portal hypertension, chronic infection and auto-immune disorders. In these patients scintigraphy shows a large active spleen with function increased in proportion to the size.

(b) Splenic infiltration – the spleen may be enlarged as a result of infiltration with pathological tissue, eg amyloid, mucopolysaccharidoses, lipidoses, glycogen storage disease. In these cases scintigraphy shows generalized splenic enlargement with function that is relatively depressed in relation to the size of the organ.

(c) Splenic masses – mass lesions arising within the spleen may present clinically with splenic enlargement. Colloid scintigraphy will detect the presence of one or more mass lesions within the spleen but will not discriminate between cysts, tumours, abscesses, haematomas or infarcts (Figs. 11.3, 11.4).

The spleen in lymphoma Detecting the presence or absence of splenic infiltration in patients with lymphoma is a problem which has not yet been solved by imaging methods. However, a number of points can be addressed by scintigraphy – the size of the spleen, the level of activity and the presence of mass lesions.

In patients with Hodgkin's lymphoma, the presence of a normal-sized and normally-functioning spleen does not rule out lymphomatous infiltration, while in other patients with Hodgkin's disease, hypersplenism (an enlarged active spleen) may exist in the absence of infiltration. This is rarely the case in non-Hodgkin's lymphoma where enlarged spleens are almost inevitably involved with tumour, and show relatively reduced function on scintigraphy. Mass

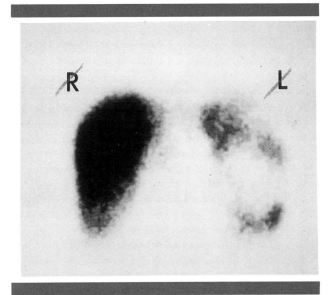

Fig. 11.3 **Large mass lesion in the spleen confirmed as cystic on computed tomography.**

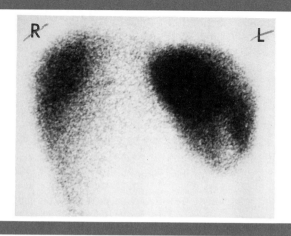

Fig. 11.4 **Posterior oblique colloid image after abdominal trauma showing a laceration in the inferior tip of the spleen.**

lesions in the spleen are a relatively rare manifestation of disease.

Hyposplenism Progressive splenic atrophy with resulting hyposplenism is a recognized feature of inflammatory bowel disease but occurs rather more frequently in adult patients with coeliac disease. Patients with diminished splenic function are at risk of increased morbidity from infection with pneumococci or other capsulated bacteria, and also malaria. Appropriate prophylactic measures can be taken once the presence of hyposplenism is recognized. The size of the spleen correlates fairly well with splenic function as measured by the rate of clearance of heat damaged red cells from the circulation (Robinson et al 1980). Scintigraphy using colloid or denatured red cells provides a convenient method for measuring the size of small spleens which may be difficult to assess by ultrasound or CT.

Some children with sickle-cell disease develop functional asplenia, ie profound hyposplenism in the presence of a spleen which is of normal size or enlarged. In these patients the splenic function is mirrored in the reduced uptake of radiocolloid or denatured red cells by the spleen, indicating the incapacity of the spleen to carry out its normal trapping function. This may be due to blockage of splenic sinusoids by clumps of sickled cells causing arteriovenous shunting of splenic blood. In some patients splenic function has been restored following transfusion with normal red cells.

Gallium scintigraphy

The technique of gallium scintigraphy is described in Chapter 9. The spleen is normally visualized on gallium images of the upper abdomen although uptake per unit volume is less than that in the liver. A generalized increase in gallium uptake in the spleen is seen in lymphomatous infiltration and in splenic enlargement due to chronic infection. Gallium may be particularly helpful in distinguishing between splenic abscesses and infarcts which may show similar appearances on CT and ultrasound.

Labelled platelets

Initial observations have suggested that the speed and intensity of uptake of autologous platelets labelled with ^{111}In can be related to hyperactivity of the spleen in patients with idiopathic thrombocytopenic purpura. The use of labelled platelet imaging of the spleen to aid the decision of whether or not to proceed with splenectomy has been proposed but at this stage the application is speculative.

REFERENCES

Dacie JV, Lewis SM 1975 Practical Haematology. Churchill Livingstone, London

Roberts JG, Wisbey ML, Newcombe RC, Baum M, Leach KG 1976 Prediction of human spleen size by computer analysis of splenic scintigrams. British Journal of Radiology **49**: 151 − 155

Robinson PJ, Bullen AW, Hall R, Brown RC, Baxter P, Losowsky MS 1980 Splenic size and function in adult coeliac disease. British Journal of Radiology **53**: 532 − 537

Index

Abscess, 54, 59, 105
  paracolic, 106
  pelvis, 106
  perinephric, 106
  subphrenic, 106
Absorption, 80
Achalasia, 9
Acute cholecystitis, 42
  cholangiography, 43
  cholecystogram, 43
  interpretation, 44
  pitfalls in
    interpretation, 46
  rationale for
    investigation, 43
  scintigraphic
    technique, 44
  ultrasound, 44
Ambulatory pH recording, 6
Amyloidosis, 64
Antibodies, 96
Atypical chest pain, 7, 8
Autonomic neuropathy, 89

Bacterial overgrowth, 83, 84
Bile acid, 82
  bacterial overgrowth, 83
  cholecystectomy, 83
  diarrhoea, 83
  idiopathic, 82
  malabsorption, 82, 84
  terminal ileum, 82
  vagotomy, 82
Bile reflux, 31
  flatulent dyspepsia, 32

post peptic ulcer
    surgery, 31
  reflux positive, 34
  reproducibility, 35
  sensitivity, 35
  total gastrectomy, 32
Biliary atresia, 37
Biliary leaks, 37, 39
Binder test, 17
Blind loop, 85
Breath tests, 84
Budd–Chiari syndrome, 52,
    65

Carcinoma
  colon, 98
  pancreas, 98
  stomach, 98
Cholangiocarcinoma, 60
Cholestyramine, 83
Chronic active hepatitis, 64
Cirrhosis, 54, 61, 62, 68, 72
Coeliac disease, 85, 134
Colloid scintigram – see Liver
    colloid scintigram
Colloid shift, 68
Columnar lined
    oesophagus, 8, 9
Condensed image, 12
Congestive heart failure, 87
Constipation, 89
Crohn's disease, 85, 87, 105

Diabetes, 8

Diarrhoea, 23, 89
Dicopac®, 81
Dilated bile ducts, 54
Dumping syndrome, 22
Duplication cysts, 94
Dysphagia, 7

Ectopic gastric mucosa, 91
Effective dose equivalent, 2

Functional gastric
       disorders, 23
Fundoplication, 8

⁶⁷Gallium citrate, 112
   sensitivity, 114
Gallstones, 42
Gastrectomy (Vitamin B12
       absorption), 80
Gastric emptying, 22
   data acquisition, 25
   detection efficiency, 25
   dumping, 26
   gastrectomy, 27
   liquid emptying, 25
   normal results, 26
   overlap, 29
   peak volume, 26
   processing the data, 26
   rapid emptying, 22
   solid meal, 25
   stasis, 23, 26, 27
   t¹/₂, 26
Gastric plication, 24
Gastric surgery, 3, 85
Gastro-oesophageal
       reflux, 17
Gastrointestinal bleeding, 91,
       116
   abnormal patterns, 124
   arteriography, 116
   clinical correlations, 127

colloid technique, 117
comprehensive
       approach, 126
correlation with
       arteriography, 126
normal appearances, 118,
       123
red cell technique, 121
scintigraphy, 116
volume of blood, 126
Glycogen storage disease, 64
Granulocytes, 107
Granulomatous hepatitis, 64

Haemangiomas, 59, 61
Haematemesis, 116
Hepatic adenomas, 59
Hepatic perfusion index, 71
Hepatitis, 62
Hepatobiliary studies, 31
Hepatomegaly, 68
HIDA
   bile acid, 33
   bilirubin levels, 33
   jaundiced patients, 33
   peak biliary excretion, 33
   protocols, 33
Hypernephroma, 106, 114

Idiopathic thrombocytopenic
       purpura, 135
Ileal resection, 84
Ileocolic fistula, 85
Infiltration of lymphatics of
       the colon, 87
Inflammatory bowel
       disease, 84, 105
Intestinal transit, 88
Intraduct stones, 32
Intrinsic factor, 80
Irradiation of the bowel, 84
Irritable bowel
       syndrome, 89

Index

Jaundice, 36
  computerized
    tomography, 36
  obstructive jaundice, 65
  transhepatic
    cholangiography, 36
  ultrasound, 36
Jejunal diverticula, 85

Leucocytes – *see*
    Radiolabelled
    leucocytes
Leukaemias, 106
Leukaemic liver
    infiltration, 65
Liver blood flow, 53, 69
  choice of tracer, 70
  curve analysis, 70
  diffuse liver disease, 72
  first pass techniques, 70
  metastatic disease, 71
  portal hypertension, 70
  portal vein occlusion, 72
  portosystemic shunts, 72
  technique, 71
Liver colloid scintigram, 49,
    58
  abscesses, 59
  ascites, 53
  benign tumours, 59
  blood volume, 59
  Budd-Chiari Syndrome
  bone marrow activity, 53
  carcinoma, 60, 64
  cholangiocarcinomas, 59
  colloid shift, 54
  costal margins, 51
  cysts, 58, 59, 61
  diffuse liver disease, 53,
    64, 67
  extraction efficiency, 49,
    53
  fatty liver, 64
  fibrosis, 58, 59

  focal liver lesions, 61
  focal nodular
    hyperplasia, 60
  gallbladder fossa, 54
  hepatitis, 62
  hepatoma, 59, 60, 66
  heterogeneous uptake, 52,
    68
  image processing, 55
  left-to-right lobe ratio, 54
  liver masses, 54, 58
  lung uptake of colloid, 54
  metastases, 56, 57
  motion correction, 55
  particle size, 50
  primary tumours, 59
  sensitivity, 50
  shape, 51
  size, 51
  SPET, 55
Liver microsphere
    angiography, 74
Liver transplant, 39
Lymphangiectasia, 85
Lymphoma, 65, 85, 106, 114,
    133

Malabsorption, 84
Meckel's diverticulum, 91
Melaena, 116
Metastases, 56, 57, 59, 68, 73
Milk scan, 20
Motility,
  refer to individual
    organs,
  small intestinal and
    colonic, 88
Myelofibrosis, 65

Neonatal hepatitis, 37
Obesity, 24
Objectives of imaging, 1
Odynophagia, 7

Oesophagus, 6
  motility, 7, 9, 13
  obstruction, 7
  oesophagitis, 6, 8, 32
  reflux, 9
  reflux test, 17
  sclerotherapy, 8
  transit test, 9
  ulceration, 16, 17
Oral contraceptives, 66

Pancreatic insufficiency, 85
Pernicious anaemia, 80
Polycythaemia rubra
      vera, 66
Polysplenia syndrome, 131
Post-operative sepsis, 106
Primary liver tumours, 59
  adenoma, 59
  carcinoma, 60
  focal nodular
      hyperplasia, 60
  haemangioma, 59
Protein-losing
      enteropathy, 87
Protein loss, 87
Proximal gastric
      vagotomy, 27
PUO, 106
Pus, 106

Radiation dose, 2
Radioimmunoscintigraphy, 96
  anti-cancer
      chemotherapy, 96
  CEA, 96
  monoclonal antibodies, 98
  radionuclides, 98
  sensitivity, 100
  skin test, 98
  staging, 96
  tomography, 99
  uptake, 99

Radiolabelled
      leucocytes, 107
  ^{111}In, 107
  abscess, 108
  faecal excretion, 112
  hepatobiliary
      excretion, 110
  HMPAO, 109
  inflammatory bowel
      disease, 108, 110, 111
Reflux oesophagitis, 6
Roux-en-y reconstruction, 31

Sarcoidosis, 107
Schilling test, 81
SeHCAT, 83
Sickle-cell disease, 134
Solitary liver lesion, 61
Sphincter of Oddi
      stenosis, 32
Spleen
  abscesses, 135
  accessory, 131
  asplenia, 134
  colloid scintigraphy, 129
  denatured red cells, 129
  hypersplenism, 132
  hyposplenism, 134
  infarcts, 135
  infiltration, 132
  labelled platelets, 135
  lymphoma, 133
  masses, 132, 133
  size, 53, 130, 133
  trauma, 131
Spleen/liver uptake ratio, 62
Splenic blood flow, 53
Steatorrhoea, 85
Sucralfate oesophageal
      study, 16
Systemic sclerosis, 8

Transfer dysphagia, 7

Index

Triolein absorption, 84
Truncal vagotomy, 27
Tuberculosis, 106
Tumour imaging – *see*
    Antibodies

Ulcerative colitis, 89, 105

Viral hepatitis, 62
Vitamin B12, 80

White blood cells – *see*
    Radiolabelled
    leucocytes